the
Illness
Experience

To Lucia Giovanna Tavano
who understands the illness experience

and

to those who helped us "through."
To those who listened as we were filled with
excitement, with frustration, with fatigue,
and with the struggles of learning.

Thank you.

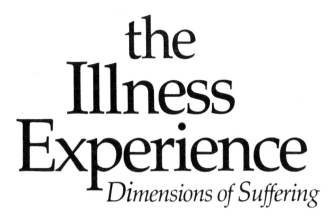

the Illness Experience

Dimensions of Suffering

Edited by
Janice M. Morse • Joy L. Johnson

 SAGE PUBLICATIONS
The International Professional Publishers
Newbury Park London New Delhi

For information address:

 SAGE Publications, Inc.
2455 Teller Road
Newbury Park, California 91320

SAGE Publications Ltd.
6 Bonhill Street
London EC2A 4PU
United Kingdom

SAGE Publications India Pvt. Ltd.
M-32 Market
Greater Kailash I
New Delhi 110 048 India

Printed in the United States of America

Library of Congress Cataloging-in-Publication Data

Main entry under title:

The Illnss experience : dimensions of suffering / [editors] Janice M.
    Morse, Joy L. Johnson.
        p.   cm.
    Includes bibliographical references and index.
    ISBN 0-8039-4053-X (c). — ISBN 0-8039-4054-8 (p)
    1. Sick—Psychology. 2. Sick—Family relationships.
3. Adjustment (Psychology) 4. Sick—Case studies. I. Morse,
Janice M. II. Johnson, Joy L.
    [DNLM: 1. Adaptation, Psychological. 2. Attitude to Health.
3. Disease—psychology. 4. Family—psychology. 5. Patients—
psychology. 6. Social Adjustment. W 85 I29]
R726.5.I45 1991
616'.001'9—dc20
DNLM/DLC   90-9226
for Library of Congress   CIP

FIRST PRINTING, 1991

Sage Production Editor: Diane S. Foster

Contents

Preface

We had frequently been told that beginning graduate students *should not* or *could not* use qualitative methods for their research. We were told that for first research projects students do not have the creativity, the skills, the ability, or the necessary confidence to conduct worthwhile qualitative work. It is said that qualitative research is too unstructured, too difficult, and requires too much theoretical knowledge for a beginning research student to develop anything worthwhile in the short time—a year—they are expected to conduct research.

These folks were wrong. Rather than being disappointed and frustrated, we have been awed at the quality of these students' projects, of their limitless creativity, and of the power and significance of the resulting research. We believe that publishing these results as 15 page articles would be so restrictive that much would be lost and that this loss would limit the impact of the research. Publishing these articles in separate journals would also limit the ability of the reader to compare and contrast the divergent experiences of patients and their relatives as they lived through nightmarish experiences with illness and the health care system.

Why has our experience been different? Are these students exceptional? Perhaps. But the other aspect that was different from the usual social science graduate student's experience is that we used the hard science "laboratory" method as a work environment. Students did not "go off" and work on their theses alone, making an appointment with their advisor every few weeks. Rather, all of the students worked within a confined laboratory space alongside a research faculty. This work environment resulted in an intensive training experience. All of these students were intimately aware of the work of the faculty and of each other; formal and informal seminars and brainstorming sessions were held regularly and frequently occurred spontaneously. This environment enabled the more seasoned students to assist those at an earlier stage of their research, which actually eased the burden for the faculty; and because the faculty could observe students on a day-to-day basis, crises and serious errors or detours were more likely to be detected and circumvented. All members of the group were intimately aware of each other's work; consequently, all the projects were, in a sense, a composite of the entire research group's work. This book is an example of the results of such efforts.

Each chapter in this book may be used as a "stand alone" example of grounded theory, as an example of substantive theory. Each chapter may be used by graduate students using grounded theory as an example of *writing* grounded theory—and how the styles and the techniques of writing may vary. By considering each study as "data," the book as a whole may be used as a preliminary tool to discuss the development of formal theory, of which the final chapter is a beginning attempt. When used in this way, this volume may be considered a beginning level graduate text.

This book was also created for the undergraduate student. For several years, we have been concerned about the lack of *context* in undergraduate education in the health sciences. We are concerned that young students are left to *care for* patients, often many years their senior, who are experiencing life altering, life threatening, or life ending experiences. Often, caring for these patients is the first encounter these students have with such weighty experiences. So we ask, how can young students appreciate what it is *like* to be a patient, to be dependent, to suffer, if they cannot even imagine the experience? The humanization of health care and a holistic approach to care have progressed some distance since professional attitudes allowed emotive empathy and other feelings for the caregiver in the caring relationship, and since this has occurred, it has become permissible—if not always acceptable—for professionals to cry with patients. But there is still a gap, and communication classes are still teaching knee-jerk responsiveness, for instance, if the patient feels ____, then respond ____. For some time, this gap has been partially filled by students reading lay accounts in the literature, such as Lear's *Heart Sounds* (1980) or Stinsons's *Long Dying of Baby Andrew* (1979/1983), in order to glimpse into the patient's or the relative's experience. However, as grounded theory is developed from more than one person's experience, it reveals a higher level of abstractness and contributes to the generation of theory, and it is more generalizable than popular accounts. It is hoped that this volume will be used to fill the gap and to teach students *what illness is really like.*

As mentioned earlier, this research has not been developed by these students alone. First, members of their thesis committees provided substantial input. All of the students' committees were chaired or cochaired by Janice Morse. Members were

- Dr. Janice Morse (Nursing), Dr. Dianne Kieren (Family Studies), and Dr. Stacey Levine (Nursing) for Joy Johnson;
- Dr. Janice Morse (Nursing), Dr. David Cumming (Medicine), and Dr. Vangie Bergum (Nursing) for Marie Andrée Chassé;
- Dr. Janice Morse (Nursing), Dr. Paul Satoris (Educational Psychology), and Dr. Terry Davis (Nursing) for Beverley Lorencz;
- Dr. Janice Morse (Nursing), Dr. Al MacKay (Educational Psychology), and Dr. Darlene Forrest (Nursing) for Sharon Wilson;
- Dr. Janice Morse (Nursing), Dr. Fred Morrison (Family Studies), and Dr. Norah Keating (Family Studies) for Judy Norris.

Others who contributed conceptually to these works and who provided moral support were Joan Bottorff, M.Ed., M.N., Ph.D. (candidate), Julie Boddy, M.P., Gail Ewing, Ph.D., and Patricia Donahue, B.Sc. (Nursing). We are indebted to Don Wells, M.A:., who over the years has become an integral part of the research group, contributing commas and common sense and that necessary laughter. We would also like to thank Pam Ratner for her "sharp eyes" and her cogent comments, Bob Morse for his comments, and Murray Pearson for the graphics. Finally, we wish to acknowledge the support we have received from *SAGE* Publications and our editors, Mitch Allen and Christine Smedley. Research grants have been received from the Alberta Foundation for Nursing Research, the Alberta

Association of Registered Nurses, the Canadian Nurses Foundation, and a Province of Alberta Fellowship Award to Joy Johnson and a Research Scholar Award from NHRDP/MRC to Janice Morse.

References

Lear, M. W. (1980). *Heart sounds*. New York: Simon & Schuster.
Stinson, R., & Stinson, P. (1979/1983). *The long dying of baby Andrew*. Boston: Little, Brown.

1

Understanding the Illness Experience

JANICE M. MORSE
JOY L. JOHNSON

What is it like to be ill? Our ability to imagine the illness experience and to empathize with those who are ill is severely limited. Until one is actually in the patient role, it is difficult to place oneself in the position of a patient. In fact being a patient is such an unexpectedly disturbing experience that even physicians who have worked with the ill on a daily basis have written accounts of their experiences as a patient in an attempt to "jolt" their peers into a new kind of awareness when interacting with patients. Books such as Sacks' *A Leg To Stand On* (1984) have become invaluable sources for medical and health care professionals. These books, however, usually describe the experiences of one person, they are often considered limited, and therefore have been dismissed as biography, merely describing extraordinary personal experiences.

A second source for those seeking to understand the illness experience is the relatively recent research literature. Medical sociologists have examined such aspects of the illness experience as physician-patient relationships, discourse relating to the illness experience, the social ramifications of lifestyle (such as stigma), illness trajectories, and the patient role. Anthropologists, have also contributed to such research by exploring the relationship between illness and culture; for example, by examining explanatory models of illness, health practices, customs, and behaviors, including ritual and traditional healing practices. Psychologists have contributed by exploring health beliefs and behaviors, such as noncompliance and coping with illness. Despite this emerging body of literature the understanding of illness behavior remains largely fragmented and in its infancy (Conrad, 1990).

For many years, the education of health professionals has focused on *disease* and *treatment processes* rather than on illness *per se* (Kleinman, 1988). Practitioners utilizing a disease model as the basis for their practice have tended to focus on pathological processes. This has resulted in an emphasis on the physiological aspects of disease rather than on the emotional and psychological responses to illness. Consequently, behavioral responses to illness have been considered beyond the purview of medical science and are still not included in the curricula of many programs that prepare physicians. The medical model necessitates that the practitioner focus solely on the disease rather than on the patient, and on the cell and tissue rather than on the person. That this view has been widely accepted in the medical world is evidenced by such jargon as the "the kidney in bed four" or the "gall bladder down the hall." The patient is treated as a disease rather than as a *person with a disease*. Clearly, the reduction of persons to their physical parts does not ensure the humane and effective care of patients.

On the other hand, the illness perspective provides a more comprehensive view, incorporating individuals and their families as they make sense of, respond to, cope with, and adapt to symptoms and disabilities (Kleinman, 1988). The illness experience does not necessarily presuppose the presence of disease. Therefore, an understanding of disease processes and treatment is a necessary but not a sufficient condition for the humane and effective care of patients. The illness perspective overcomes the limitations inherent in the medical model and ensures that patients are treated as *persons* and not as objects. The illness perspective integrates the mind-body dichotomy within the social context, acknowledging that people are more than physiological entities.

Since Parsons (1951) first introduced his classical theories on the sick role, many authors have described aspects of the illness experience. Despite the fact that a comprehensive illness model could provide insights for health care professionals as well as a basis for the planning and implementation of care, a satisfactory model has yet to be developed. Ideally, such a model should

    (1) incorporate the entire duration of the illness experience, beginning with the onset of symptoms,
    (2) allow for the expression of the dynamic nature of illness,
    (3) be based on the patient's perspective,

(4) identify the similarities that arise from illness, rather than the underlying disease,

(5) incorporate the entire context of the illness into the model, and

(6) be developed inductively without implying or imposing a previously developed model.

As stated, the first requirement to understanding the illness experience is that the entire experience should be incorporated into the model. Illness does not begin when the individual first comes into contact with the physician or the emergency room. Rather, there is a significant period of decision making and self-treatment which is aimed at controlling symptoms and to healing one's-self (Dingwall, 1976). Often in this period there is extensive consultation with others and the use of over-the-counter medications and lay therapies.

Second, as the course of illness changes dramatically, occasionally even from moment to moment throughout the course of disease, the model needs to allow for changes in the patient's condition, changes in therapy, and changes in care requirements. The needs of a patient at one point in time may not be relevant to the next; consequently the model must permit versatility and flexibility.

Third, theories of illness must be developed from the patient's perspective rather than from the perspective of the health care provider, social worker, or significant others. Only by eliciting thick descriptions of the patient's experiences with illness can an understanding of the patient's needs be developed and anticipated. Inferring the patient's needs from the perspective of the caregiver is arrogant and paternalistic, yet we continue to discount the patient's report of symptoms (e.g., by discounting the patient's pain) and insist instead that the caregiver is best informed about the ill person's needs and wishes.

The fourth requirement of an illness experience model is the need to identify behavioral commonalities inherent in the illness experience. We know that behavior is patterned and the course of illness follows a distinct path regardless of the underlying pathology, yet to date these commonalities have not been explicated.

Fifth, the model must incorporate a holistic perspective, including the significant others and environmental and contextual factors. The ill person does not exist in isolation, even if ironically the health care system isolates the patient. The patient has had a life before being institutionalized, interacts with other patients, health care providers and visitors, responds to treatments, and anticipates the future; consequently, these factors cannot be ignored in the course of treatment.

Finally, a model of illness must be developed inductively, without the imposition of another model or theory on the experience. Similarly, the model or theory must fit into what is already known about the illness experience, and it must not be developed or exist in isolation from the current literature. Thus although the model will extend, clarify, or correct our present understanding of the illness experience it is unlikely that it will be revolutionary.

Qualitative methods allow for the development of models without losing any of the above characteristics. In particular, grounded theory is best suited to describing processes, allowing the necessary versatility that is required for complex phenomena such as the course of the illness experience. The remainder of this chapter will be a discussion of the research methods used to elicit the illness experience. Chapters Two through Six in this book are examples of grounded theories describing the illness experience from the perspective of those involved: either the patient or a relative. The last chapter, Chapter Seven, is a synthesis of the similarities of the illness experiences described in the five studies, and it is an attempt to develop a comprehensive model of the illness experience.

The Method of Grounded Theory

The five investigators whose studies are reported in this book all used the method of grounded theory to investigate the illness experience. The origins of grounded theory are derived from ethnography and symbolic interactionism. From ethnography, grounded theory has acquired interview methods, participant observation, and the incorporation of other sources of information such as patient records. But most significantly, the influence of symbolic interactionism gives grounded theory its distinctiveness as a method. Further, Gerhardt (1990) notes that grounded theory has been elaborated beyond symbolic interactionism and now it takes into account the methods and philosophy of phenomenology, linguistic analysis, ethnomethodology and narrative research, and biographical research.

Briefly, *symbolic interactionism* focuses on the "inner or experiential aspects of human behaviors" (Chenitz & Swanson, 1986).

Interactionists argue that individuals order their world by a process of negotiation and renegotiation; by encapsulating, recapitulating, and rehearsing. They argue that people make reflexive use of symbols, interpreting and eliciting meanings rather than simply reacting to them, that people "construct, judge and modify" themselves as social entities in relation to the meaning attributed to the situation; and finally, that "perspectives and plans emerge out of the interplay between a socially constituted self and a socially constituted environment" (Rock, 1982, p. 35). Thus perceptions of reality are fluid and constantly created according to the definitions and meanings attributed to the situation and according to the negotiated response of the self and others within the situation.

It is this essence of change and process, of constructed and negotiated perceptions of the social world as it occurs in a natural setting, that is critical to the method of grounded theory (Stern, Allen, & Moxley, 1982). As the analysis progresses, the researcher, using constant comparison, compares all pieces of data with other pieces and identifies the *core category.* The core variable is the process that (a) is central and is related to as many other categories as possible, (b) continuously occurs in the data, and (c) accounts for most of the variation (Glaser, 1978). If the core category has two or more stages, then it is called a *Basic Social Process (BSP),* and the dynamic nature of the process forces labeling using a gerund (or an "ing" word). The stages in the *BSP* should differentiate and account for the variations in behavior. If the BSP relates to a psychological process it is referred to as a *Basic Social Psychological Process (BSPP),* and if the *BSP* refers to a social structure it is referred to as a *Basic Social Structural Process (BSSP)* (Glaser, 1978; Hutchinson, 1986). These processes will be referred to in greater detail in Chapter Seven.

Doing Grounded Theory

The first step in any research project is the identification of a topic for study. This is often the most difficult task for a researcher, particularly a student, because the scope or the realm of possibilities appear limitless and the amount that is known about the topic appears comprehensive. Therefore, the possibility of identifying a topic about which *little* is known seems remote. Thus rather than approaching the area through the library, we recommend that students identify areas or topics about which they *are interested.* Often this requires some self-examination: Students should become aware of what they find fascinating, of the types of articles they find themselves reading when leafing through journals for other articles, and topics that they often find themselves thinking about. When these areas have been identified they should narrow the topic by discussing the area with others and by looking in the library to find out what is known. Although Glaser and Strauss (1967) and Charmaz (1990) recommend doing a literature search later in the research process in order to reduce the risk of "driving" the research with concepts that have already been identified, we recommend that in order to prevent the "reinvention of the wheel" the student must first do a literature search and then "bracket" the knowledge (i.e., set it aside) and later in the investigation return to the library to link findings with the work of others.

Grounded theory questions usually have distinct characteristics. The questions themselves may suggest a process. Unlike phenomenological questions—in which the *meaning* and the *lived experience* of the participant are important, or ethnography, which may describe or interpret the informant's perspective—grounded theory is more likely to address issues such as "what is going on here?"

Having refined the question, prepared the proposal, selected a setting, and obtained appropriate ethical clearances (see Field & Morse, 1985), the next step is to select participants to interview. The purposeful selection of informants is crucial to the success of the study. Informants *must* have the qualities of a "good informant" (that is, be willing to participate, be knowledgeable about the topic, be articulate, and have time to be interviewed) (see Morse, 1986); otherwise, the interview data will be less than optimal and the number of participants will have to be increased to obtain saturation (i.e., until no new data appear). Increasing the number of participants increases the time required by the investigator as well as the research costs for transcribing interviews. As informants who *are going through* an experience may not have had the time or the energy to *make sense* of the experience, it is recommended that the first informants should be chosen from those who have passed through the experience. By hearing the entire story from beginning to end from several participants, common patterns or critical incidents will become evident to the investigator. After discovering the common patterns and critical incidents the next phase in sampling is to find informants who are presently experiencing those various phases in order to confirm or refute emerging hypotheses, to address specific questions, or to expand on certain points. The problem with following informants through an experience and interviewing them in a prospective fashion is that many details may only be apparent to the investigator in retrospect, and the investigator may spend a longer time than necessary in the period of "bewilderment."

Unfortunately, it is not always possible to identify or choose a good informant before inviting the informant to be in the study. Often the investigator must use participants who have been referred by physicians or other caregivers or who have responded to advertisements. In these cases it may be necessary to use secondary selection (Morse, 1991), that is, to determine if the participant will be retained in the study during or at the end of the first interview.

Grounded theory interviews usually start with an open-ended question such as "Tell me about. . . . " The purpose is to elicit the informant's "story" with as few prompts as possible. Informants usually tell their stories in chronological order; however, the researcher must be aware that there may be several stories imbedded in one event, and these stories may be told to meet the participant's perceived understanding of what the researcher wants to know. Thus, if the researcher is a physician then the informant will tell the story in a medical "manner," with details of symptoms, treatments, and medications—as one would normally give a physician a history—but omitting significant data on feelings; whereas if the interviewer were a lay person the story would be quite different. If the researcher believes that the story is being told on the wrong level, then it will be necessary to interrupt in order to elicit the type of information required.

Transcription and analysis of the interviews begins immediately following the interview, and there is a responsive interaction between the collection of data and the analysis, with the interviews directing the coding and vice versa. In grounded theory "in vivo" codes are used, that is rather than using known concepts or variable labels as codes (such as "social support" or "coping") labels are taken directly from the interview using the language that the informants themselves use (Strauss, 1987). Thus the researcher examines and codes the transcript line by line, highlighting important passages and creating theoretical memos (i.e., notes, insights, comparisons, summaries, questions) during the task. The next level of coding involves performing content analysis by selecting passages or significant

portions of the text and copying these pieces onto separate categories of similar text. This process simplifies the task of constant
comparison, of comparing each quotation with all other pieces in
order to note the similarities and differences of examples within each
category. The final step is to identify the linkages between the
categories by comparing and contrasting the conditions and consequences of the relationship between the concepts.

The process of analysis is highly interactive between the emerging
research and the interviews. As new ideas become evident the
interviews with the informants are redirected to elicit new information. In these interviews the researcher probes for more information
if the researcher considers a part of the data thin or has unanswered
questions about certain aspects. At this point the researcher confirms
developing hypotheses with secondary informants, and if necessary
may even "change direction," following a lead by interviewing a
different group of participants.

As greater understanding of the research topic is obtained, the core
variable or the *BSP* may become evident. As stated, when the core
variable has two or more stages the term *BSPP* or *BSSP* is used. In
the analytic process of delineating the stages and the characteristics
of each stage, diagraming and mapping are used extensively. These
processes enable increased levels of abstractness and clarify the
development of the theory.

One strategy of diagraming is the construction of typologies
(Glaser, 1978). The researcher first identifies two variables or emerging concepts that appear to contribute to the variance in the phenomena and, using a 2×2 matrix, explores the effects of the presence
or absence of each variable in combinations. For example, Johnson
used a 2×2 matrix to exemplify the relationship between the
informants' perceived needs and the amount of perceived support.
The use of a 2×2 matrix helped to clarify the relationship between
these two variables and to clarify important distinctions.

In the descriptions of processes, most of these authors have
developed models that illustrate the relationships of the various
variables and concepts or the process of moving through an experience. Chassé described an extensive pathway that participants use
when trying to determine if they are ill, which she has labeled
establishing the boundaries of normalcy, and Lorencz developed a
flowchart depicting the process of *becoming ordinary,* illustrating
the struggle that people diagnosed with schizophrenia anticipate in

the period prior to their hospital discharge. Other authors have used lists to compare characteristics of various attributes. For example, Johnson used a list to compare the factors that affected the informants' view of the future and using this list she contrasted those who had a positive attitude with those who had elected to "wait and see."

Are Grounded Theory Studies Reliable and Valid?

In grounded theory, reliability is established by ensuring the appropriateness of the sample and the adequacy of the data (Morse, 1986). The use of a purposeful sample ensures appropriateness. The sample should be selected according to the theoretical needs of the study, the willingness of the participants to participate, and the ability of the informants to describe their insights. Thus the sample is representative of the phenomena under study rather than the population in general.

Adequacy of the data is determined by the amount of data obtained rather than by the number of subjects participating in the study. Adequacy is obtained when the data are saturated (i.e., when no new data are obtained, and when all aspects of the phenomena are richly described). In other words, adequacy is achieved when the theory is valid and complete.

How Generalizable is Grounded Theory?

When the theory has been developed from a relatively small number of participants it is often assumed that the theory is in no way generalizable; however, it should be noted that grounded theory does not attempt to quantify attributes and therefore generalizability acquires a slightly different meaning. The generalizability that is referred to here is *theoretical generalizability,* that is, the theory or the model that is developed should be applicable to others who experience the same conditions or illnesses. Theoretical generalizability may be extended even further as the substantive theory may give rise to formal theory. That is, by linking the theories with the literature and by linking grounded theories it is possible to develop a generalizable theory of illness, and it is the beginning of such a theory that is developed in the final chapter.

This volume consists of five studies completed by graduate students as a part of their masters' degrees. The questions addressed by

Johnson in the first study were "What is the process of adjustment that an individual experiences following a myocardial infarction?" and "In what ways do the experiences of men and women differ following myocardial infarction?"

In the second study, Chassé addressed the question "What are the experiences of women who undergo a hysterectomy?" In her study she examined the physical and psychosocial issues that women attempt to resolve when they undergo this surgical procedure and the strategies that women use when attempting to adjust.

In the third study, Lorencz asked, "What are the perceptions of adult chronic schizophrenics during planned transition from the hospital to the community?" In this study she explored the primary concerns of chronic schizophrenics who are anticipating returning to the community and their descriptions of leaving a psychiatric care facility.

Although it may be argued that *abortion* is not an illness, the fourth study, by Norris, is included because abortion is treated as a surgical procedure in hospitals. Certainly the findings generated by the question "What is the social-psychological experience of mothers who consent for their daughter's abortions?" reveal acute distress, a lack of support, and an unmet need to talk about the experience with a neutral listener.

Finally, Wilson described the husband's experiences of living with a wife who undergoes chemotherapy treatment for cancer. She explicated the husband's response to his wife's situation and examined the strategies that the husband found most helpful when living through this "unrelenting nightmare."

These diverse studies on the illness experience and the suffering of patients and their families have similarities despite the different diseases, treatments, and prognoses. It is these patterns that are associated with "just being ill," of being a patient, or of being a relative that are drawn together in the final chapter of this book. Two factors appear to make a wise practitioner: the understanding of the individual illness experience and the recognition of patterns and common experiences that are a part of human responses to illness. The acquisition of both these levels of knowledge greatly facilitates the provision of expert care, whether in the form of counseling by psychologists, care by physicians or nurses, or support by neighbors.

Although this book only begins to "scratch the surface" of the illness experience, it is a start. We recognize that the synthesis, or the meta-analysis, of the five studies in this book represents preliminary work and that there is much work to be done in the development of the *Illness-Constellation Model* which is presented in the final chapter.

Many of the experiences described in the following chapters are very moving and we make no apologies for their poignancy. We recognize the intensity of these experiences and that these experiences may not be representative of the entire range of responses in the illness experience and that an individual's experiences with illness may differ from those described in this text, either reflecting more suffering or involving different problems or concerns. Further research is required if these differences are to be fully understood. We are grateful to the informants whose willingness to share their experiences openly allowed us a new look at the illness experience.

References

Charmaz, K. (1990). "Discovering" chronic illness: Using grounded theory. *Social Science & Medicine, 30,* 1161-1172.

Chenitz, W. C., & Swanson, J. M. (1986). *From practice to grounded theory.* Menlo Park, CA: Addison-Wesley.

Conrad, P. (1990). Qualitative research on chronic illness: A commentary on methods and conceptual development. *Social Science & Medicine, 30,* 1257-1263.

Dingwall, R. (1976). *Aspects of illness.* New York: St. Martin's Press.

Field, P. A., & Morse, J. M. (1985). *Nursing research: The application of qualitative approaches.* London: Croom Helm.

Glaser, B. G. (1978). *Theoretical sensitivity.* Mill Valley, CA: The Sociology Press.

Glaser, B. G., & Strauss, A. L. (1967). *The discovery of grounded theory: Strategies for qualitative research.* New York: Aldine.

Gerhardt, U. (1990). Qualitative research on chronic illness: The issue and the story. *Social Science & Medicine, 30*(11), 1149-1159.

Hutchinson, S. (1986). Grounded theory: The method. In P. L. Munhall & C. J. Oiler (Eds.), *Nursing research: A qualitative perspective* (pp. 111-130). East Norfolk, CT: Appleton-Century-Crofts.

Kleinman, A. (1988). *The illness narratives: Suffering, healing and the human condition.* New York: Basic Books.

Morse, J. M. (1986). Quantitative and qualitative research: Issues in sampling. In P. L. Chinn (Ed.), *Nursing research methodology: Issues and implementation* (pp. 181-194). Rockville, MD: Aspen.

Morse, J. M. (1991). Strategies for sampling. In J. Morse (Ed.), *Qualitative nursing research: A contemporary dialogue* (rev. ed.) (pp. 127-145). Newbury Park, CA: Sage.

Parsons, T. (1951). *The social system.* New York: Free Press.

Rock, P. (1982). Symbolic interaction. In R. B. Smith & P. K. Manning (Eds.), *Handbook of social science methods, Vol. 2: Qualitative methods* (pp. 33-47). Cambridge, MA: Ballinger.

Sacks, O. (1984). *A leg to stand on.* New York: Harper & Row.

Stern, P. N., Allen, L. M., & Moxley, P. A. (1982). The nurse as grounded theorist: History, process and uses. *Review Journal of Philosophy & Social Science, 7,* 200-215.

Strauss, A. L. (1987). *Qualitative analysis for social scientists.* Cambridge, UK: Cambridge University Press.

2

Learning to Live Again: The Process of Adjustment Following a Heart Attack

JOY L. JOHNSON

Feeling unwell? At what point do you consider yourself sick? And when you are sick, at what point do you call the ambulance? The process of waiting to see if the symptoms dissipate, the testing to find out what makes the symptoms worse or better can continue for several days. To admit that one requires help is to admit that the symptoms are beyond one's control. The signs and symptoms of a heart attack often begin insidiously and escalate over a period of hours. Heart attacks have a paradoxical nature. Although potentially fatal, the early signs of a heart attack mimic minor and trivial complaints. Unless the heart attack is extensive, the early symptoms may be interpreted as indigestion, the flu, a pulled muscle, or food poisoning. For example, in the following study, one participant delayed seeking medical attention for three days.

The irony of delaying treatment is caused in part by the mixed messages given to the public. On one hand, the signs and symptoms of heart attack are well publicized because it is assumed that people who recognize the combination of symptoms will seek help early. On the other hand, people are reluctant to go to hospital emergency rooms or "bother" their physicians with seemingly minor complaints. Media accounts of the health care system often give the impression that there is major concern with an overutilization of health care facilities and with the cost of

AUTHOR'S NOTE: Derived from: Johnson, J. L. (1988). *The process of adjustment following myocardial infarction.* Unpublished master's thesis, University of Alberta, Edmonton, Alberta, Canada.

This research was supported in part by the Alberta Association of Registered Nurses and the Alberta Foundation for Nursing Research.

nonurgent consultations. Furthermore, health care professionals are frequently annoyed by nonurgent consultations and become condescending toward patients with "minor" complaints. In turn, these attitudes manage to embarrass patients and ensure that they learn not to "misuse" emergency services.

The process of assessing the severity and meaning of symptoms and somatic experiences continues for patients through the acute and rehabilitative phases. It is almost as if they are constantly holding their breath, hoping that each twinge is not another heart attack. This process is not only internal, but it also includes carefully monitoring the responses of others, especially the responses of health care professionals. Spoken or unspoken, implicit or explicit indications of their progress are used by heart attack patients to gauge their recovery. Seemingly minor signs of progress such as looks of relief from health care professionals, and successfully achieving milestones such as walking a flight of stairs, provide concrete evidence of progress for heart attack patients. But is this enough? Unfortunately it is not enough because the mixed messages continue: "You are well enough to do without a cardiac monitor, but it must be attached when you exercise." "You are as good as new, but take it easy for six weeks." "You are recovering well, but keep taking your medication." Heart attack victims' lives are plagued by uncertainties. They must continue to test their abilities until they once again trust their bodies. The stages of the adjustment process following a heart attack and the strategies that men and women use to negotiate these stages are described in the following chapter.

Despite the substantial volume of research literature in the field of cardiac rehabilitation, the process of adjustment that an individual experiences following a myocardial infarction (MI) is not very well understood. To date, investigators have focused on specific aspects of rehabilitation, such as the incidence of anxiety and depression and the frequency with which individuals return to work. The importance of the individual's perceptions of his or her recovery following an MI has not been acknowledged. Consequently, research findings in the field of cardiac rehabilitation offer a fragmented understanding of the process of adjustment experienced by individuals following a heart attack.

The majority of research studies in the field of cardiac rehabilitation have focused on the male patient. There has been a failure to acknowledge that the female experience may be different from that of the male. There are strong indications that the experiences of men and women following a heart attack are different, yet these differences have not been fully explored.

The treatment of the MI patient has been aptly described as a "Tower of Babel" in which each group of health professionals uses a different model to assess and treat the patient (Bar-On, 1986). This situation is further confused as the patient inevitably has yet another perspective. Therefore, a qualitative study was conducted in order to gain an understanding of men's and women's experiences following an MI. Interviews with 14 individuals (7 of whom were female) who had experienced an MI were the major source of data.[1]

The Initial Stages of the Adjustment Process

Regaining Control

The process of adjustment following a heart attack begins with the onset of symptoms and involves a struggle to regain control. Control has been described in a variety of ways. In this study it was found that the core category, *regaining control,* is a complex process which involves three dimensions: regaining a sense of predictability, self-determination, and independence (see Figure 2.1).[2]

A *sense of predictability,* the first dimension of control, involves the perception that any responses that are made will have some impact on the outcome of a person's life. This perception is based on an individual's ability to use past experiences to foretell the immediate future. Predictability is an aspect of control that is often taken for granted. Not having to "think twice" before climbing a flight of stairs is an example of predictability. An individual is normally able to engage in such a task knowing that he or she will arrive at the top of the stairs. A heart attack imposes physical and psychological restrictions on a person's life. It introduces a sense of uncertainty which, in turn, diminishes predictability. The heart attack victim must regain a sense of predictability before a sense of personal control can be fully regained.

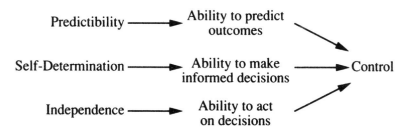

Figure 2.1. The Dimensions of Personal Control

Self-determination is the second dimension of control that is affected by the experience of a heart attack. Self-determination involves decisional control: the power to understand what is happening and to make autonomous decisions. A heart attack is a frightening and unfamiliar event. Heart attack victims typically have little understanding of heart disease and its treatment. A lack of understanding about what is occurring to one's body undermines an individual's sense of power and control, and the victim must make sense of the heart attack before he or she is able to regain a sense of control.

Similarly, one's *independence,* the third dimension of control, is threatened by a heart attack. The ability to act on decisions is disrupted by limitations, both real and perceived. The victim is no longer able to trust his or her abilities and therefore must rely on others for support. As the heart attack victim regains a sense of independence he or she is able to regain a sense of control.

Clearly, a heart attack not only has implications for one's physiological well-being, it has an impact upon every aspect of one's life. All of the informants in this study said that they believed the heart is central to life and vitality; consequently the occurrence of a heart attack threatened every aspect of the informants' lives, threatened their very beings:

> Your heart is central to your life. Your heart does the most. . . . It seems if anything happens to your heart, it's like a big attack on you. I think that's why they call it a heart attack instead of a heart problem.

The loss of control experienced as a result of the heart attack is often devastating, and the struggle to regain control is frustrating. The informants in this study described the heart attack as a threat to their "whole" lives. They felt "fragmented" as a result of the heart attack, and they experienced a total lack of control:

> It wasn't the right time. It could have waited until later when I was ready to say it could happen. I had my life figured out, and I didn't want this stupid thing coming in there and telling me what to do. . . . It popped into my life, and it had no business being there because I hadn't willed it.
>
> I don't know what to do. I do not like to be adrift at the mercy of other people telling me what to do. I want to know what's going on. I want to play a role in what's going on.

The process of adjustment was not completed until the informants were able to regain a sense of control.

Following a heart attack there is a process of adjustment that can last from six months to two years. Unlike transient conditions, a heart attack leaves the victim with permanent heart damage. An individual cannot fully recover following a heart attack; at best he or she will be able to compensate and adjust. The heart attack will not be forgotten and the ability to unconsciously rely on the heart will never be present to the extent that it was prior to the heart attack.

The process of adjustment following a heart attack is comprised of four interrelated stages: defending one's self, coming to terms with the event, learning to live, and living again. The process of regaining control persists throughout these four stages (see Figure 2.2). In the first stage, the heart attack victim fights to maintain control over his or her life. During the second stage, the heart attack victim struggles with a perceived loss of control. In the third stage, the heart attack victim begins the struggle to reestablish a sense of control over his or her life. Finally, if the victims are able to meet the challenge of regaining control they enter the fourth stage in the process, the stage where a sense of personal control is acquired.

Stage One: Defending Oneself

Heart attacks occur suddenly and with little warning. Not having previously experienced a heart attack, the individual is often

Regaining Control

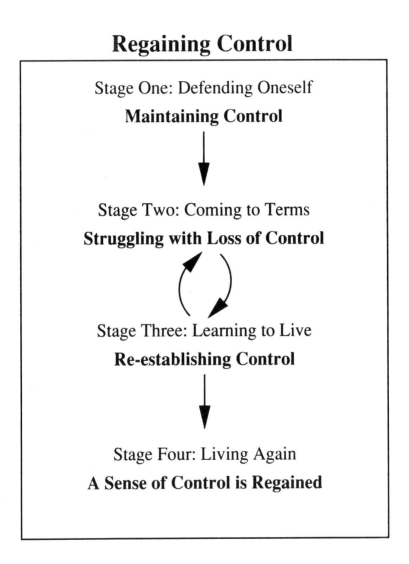

Figure 2.2. The Process of Regaining Control

confused by the presenting symptoms. Despite the severity of the initial symptoms, every attempt is made not to "give in" to the symptoms in order to maintain a sense of control. In the first stage of adjustment the individual struggles to defend him- or herself against the threatened loss of control. Three strategies are used in this first stage of adjustment: normalizing the symptoms, struggling to maintain the *status quo,* and, finally, distancing oneself.

Normalizing Symptoms

All of the informants were asked to share their stories, and all of them began the discussion of their experiences with a description of their initial symptoms. The nature and severity of the initial symptoms varied from informant to informant; however, in every case past events and experiences were used to make sense of the initial symptoms. Making sense of the symptoms involved a cognitive process of relating the presenting symptoms to previous experiences with health problems. The informants refused to consider their symptoms extraordinary; rather, attempts were made to normalize the symptoms. Consequently, decisions regarding the course of action to follow were based on this attempt to normalize the symptoms:

> I started to feel sick, and I thought, "You know, there's a lot of flu going around. I wonder if this is the flu." So I went and lay down.

> My opinion was that I've got a chest cold. I didn't believe that I was having a heart attack. My opinion was that I've got a chest cold and that was the problem. . . . So I got up to take some cough syrup.

> I've never had an experience with a heart attack, so I thought it was just a pulled chest muscle. So I stood up and inhaled, and I held my breath, and this kind of relieved it. When I let my breath out, it went back to being painful again.

The informants' attempts to normalize and treat their symptoms lasted for up to three days following their onset. If their initial conclusions about symptom etiology were disproved, the informants frequently continued to seek other causal explanations. For example, one informant who initially determined that his "heart burn" was due to stress later thought that he had the flu. This decision was made when his symptoms changed and he began to experience chills and nausea. The speed with which the initial symptoms escalated influenced the ability of the informant to continue to normalize the symptoms.

Other factors that influenced the informants' attempts to normalize the symptoms included preconceived ideas about heart attack symptomatology and etiology. In particular, three of the women in this investigation persisted in their attempts to normalize their symptoms because they believed women are not susceptible to heart attacks. In one situation this belief was held by the informant's husband. The informant believed that something serious was happening to her, and she was concerned and turned to her husband for support. Her husband assured her that there was nothing wrong. According to this informant, her husband did not believe that women could have heart attacks.

Informants who had preconceived ideas regarding the "typical" symptoms of a heart attack often prolonged their attempts to normalize their symptoms. For example, some informants believed that the hallmark of a heart attack is excruciating chest pain. Symptoms such as nausea, chills, weakness, and excessive perspiration presented a confusing picture to these individuals. Although they suspected that something serious was happening to them, they quickly dismissed the possibility of a heart attack as they believed that their symptoms did not match the typical heart attack symptoms:

> Well, not having a heart attack, no one knows anything. You hear this and that, and it's not always true. It's amazing the things you don't know. Like, when I was kneeling in front of the toilet there, throwing up my guts, all I could think of was "I must have caught the flu" or "I've got food poisoning." Like, I had no idea that was one of the signs of a heart attack. And I was never out of breath, you know. I had heard you get really short of breath. It never happened.

> I always thought with a heart attack that you get this pain in your left arm. I thought it couldn't be a heart attack, that pain wasn't there. So I think that was the classic thing that threw me.

Other informants continued their attempts to normalize symptoms because they believed that nothing terrible could possibly happen to them. They described their initial symptoms as "no big deal."

Despite the presence of serious symptoms, these informants persisted with this attitude. When asked why he persisted in this belief one informant said, "Everybody thinks these things happen to someone else, not me. Same old attitude: It won't ever get me." Attempting to normalize their symptoms provided these individuals with a mechanism to maintain a sense of control.

Struggling to Maintain the *Status Quo*

As attempts to alleviate the symptoms of "colds," "flu," "food poisoning," and "muscle pulls" fail, the individual begins to consider the possibility that something out of the ordinary may be happening to him or her; however, rather than seek assistance he or she attempts to suppress this belief. To admit that something serious is happening is to admit that one is not in control. By seeking assistance, the individual fears that his or her worst fears may be confirmed. At this point, the individual begins to struggle to maintain the *status quo*:

> I only had a slight idea what might be happening, but I thought the standard "Hey, it can't be me." So I got up and threw up once. I was getting weaker all the time. But I stayed at work for the day.

Rather than seek assistance, the informants made every attempt to ignore the possibility that something serious might be happening to them and they attempted to "carry on as usual." Endeavoring to maintain the *status quo* allowed these individuals to maintain a sense of control; however, this struggle was extremely difficult as the informants had to contend with several factors, including their own sense that something ominous was occurring and pressure from others to seek assistance. These factors created a feeling of tension in the informants, which they had to fight to overcome. Many of the informants described their efforts to persuade others that they were all right. Despite a feeling that they were not "all right," these informants often continued to deny they had a serious problem:

> [A friend] came in and said, "What's the matter with you? You look terrible. What's wrong?" And I said, "I don't feel very good." He said, "Why don't you get yourself over to the hospital?" And I said, "Just leave me alone. I'm going to finish work, and then I'm going home."

She kept on saying, "Mom, let's go to the hospital . . . you don't look good." She just thought there was something wrong with me, and I kept on saying, "Oh, it's all gone, I'm fine."

In retrospect, many of the informants recognized that to face the fact that they required help was to recognize that the situation was beyond their own control.

In addition to managing the pressure to seek assistance that was exerted by others, the informants had to contend with their own sense that "something" was happening:

I usually have a bottle of beer after work. [But] it didn't taste good. That's very strange, it always tastes good after putting in your nine hours. . . . When I get home, I usually do a crossword to get my tenseness out, and I didn't feel like that either.

I thought, "Gee, should I stop for lunch or shouldn't I? . . . I didn't have any breakfast today, maybe I'm feeling a bit hungry." So I made myself a half a sandwich. I normally make a whole sandwich, and I thought, "I wonder why."

Despite attempts to maintain the *status quo* the informants felt that something was not right. This perception was unsettling as it required the informants to recognize that something out of the ordinary was occurring.

Two factors prompted the informants to seek assistance: an exacerbation of their symptoms and the repeated urging of friends and family to seek assistance. The exacerbation of symptoms was often accompanied by a sense of impending doom, and this sense of doom forced the individual to surrender the struggle to maintain the *status quo*. The symptoms were magnified to such a degree that they could no longer be normalized. What was initially believed to be "normal" began to be viewed as "extraordinary." At this point the informants believed they had lost the capacity to fight and they realized that assistance was required:

I started throwing up, and I threw up really badly. In fact, I was down on my knees in the can, and then I thought, "I can't do this anymore." So I flopped out on the floor, and I couldn't move. I just called my husband. I said, "I'm really sick!" . . . So he called the ambulance.

It was difficult for the informants to seek help. Many of them felt caught between a desire to maintain control and the belief that they required assistance. However, as their symptoms continued to exacerbate it was difficult for the informants to ignore the increasing sense of uneasiness and the severity of the symptoms and their attempts to normalize the symptoms and maintain the *status quo* became impossible. Once it became impossible to maintain the *status quo* the informants desperately tried to ease their minds. In one situation an informant attempted to "relieve his mind" by looking for a bookmark that had the signs and symptoms of a heart attack printed on it. He believed that the bookmark would provide proof that he was all right. He enlisted his family members to help him, and with their assistance he spent half an hour searching for the bookmark. The bookmark was eventually found but it failed to rid him of his uneasiness:

> Well then, when I found the bookmark, I went through the symptoms and let's say there's five symptoms on it I could relate to myself: your chest pains, your arms going numb, you're nauseated, you're clammy. And I thought, "Well, if nothing else, we'll go up to the hospital . . . to relieve my mind."

The second factor that prompted the informants to seek assistance was the pressure exerted by their family members and friends. As the result of repeated coaxing, several informants agreed to seek assistance. In some cases the trip to the hospital or physician was not made as a result of the individual believing that he or she required assistance; rather, he or she chose to seek assistance in order to "ease the minds" of others:

> We'll go to the hospital to relieve my mind and also to relieve my wife's and family's mind. 'Cause they wanted me to go, and I kept saying, "No, there's nothing wrong. It will go away."

> And a third person told me that I was looking badly and why don't I go to the hospital. And so I walked across. They wanted me to go to the hospital, and so I said, "I'll walk across."

By choosing to seek assistance for the sake of others these individuals were able to maintain a sense of personal control.

Distancing Oneself

Once the decision to seek assistance was made the informants
were quick to act. Most of the informants in this study chose to visit
hospital emergency rooms; however, two informants visited their
general practitioners. Once professional help was solicited the informants began to ponder the severity of their situations. The sense
of severity was often reinforced by the reactions of the health care
professionals who assisted them:

> So I went to see the G. P. [General Practitioner]. The description I've given
> to people is if you've ever seen a doctor's face cloud over and they give
> you the "you're going to die, son, look" that's what I got at that point.

> The girl at the admitting desk said, "What is your problem?" And I said,
> "Well, I have pains in my chest, and my arm has sort of gone funny on
> me." . . . She immediately left to get a doctor. And within a few seconds,
> there's a doctor back, and they're getting a stretcher.

At this point, the informants began to distance themselves from
the events, symptoms, and, if possible, the reality that something had
gone terribly wrong. Many of the informants said their recollections
of the events that occurred during the initial days in the hospital were
"foggy." Rather than remain engaged in the crisis, attempts were
made to avoid the terrible reality of the symptoms and the hospital
environment. This distancing provided the informants with some
"space" away from the crisis. Through the process of distancing, the
informants disengaged themselves from the ongoing events. This, in
turn, allowed them the freedom to avoid feeling a loss of control. In
addition, distancing themselves allowed the informants an opportunity to gather their resources prior to facing the reality of a heart
attack. Distancing strategies continued until the informants were
ready to come to terms with their heart attack.

The ways in which the individuals in this study managed to
distance themselves from the "real world" varied a great deal. One
of the most common forms of distancing occurred within the first
few days of hospitalization. The informants refused to believe that
something terrible was happening to them. The result of this denial
was a sense that they were not involved in a horror-filled reality; instead, they were removed from it. Many of the informants described

the events in the emergency room and the intensive care unit as "far away" or "unreal." They were unable to keep track of time. Two informants described a sensation of living in "slow motion." Many of them said they did not feel present during the initial days or hours of hospitalization. Their bodies were present, yet they were not emotionally involved in the ongoing events. In retrospect, many of the informants believed that they used this distancing in order to protect themselves:

> At one point, though, I thought I was visiting my mother, and she was having the heart attack, and she'd been dead two years. I guess I was just trying to put it on somebody else so I wouldn't have it.

The most extreme form of distancing was experienced by a woman who was gravely ill:

> I can remember them working over me there, and it was strange. Like it really hurt and that. And then for awhile, it just seemed like I was just sitting up there watching myself have a heart attack, and it didn't bother me at all. I was just watching all these people running around working.

Although some might describe this phenomenon as an "out of body experience," it can also be viewed as an extreme form of distancing. This woman was able to effectively remove herself from the pain of a heart attack. She believed that she had partially "willed" herself to remain distanced because she was "overwhelmed" by the pain and the stress.

Even though the symptoms were controlled and the diagnosis was shared with the informant, the informants continued to use a distancing strategy. Rather than face what had happened and the uncertainty of the future many of the informants continued to distance themselves by refusing to believe that the heart attack happened or by denying the diagnosis:

> Afterwards, it didn't seem like I had a heart attack. It didn't seem real. I thought, "Somebody else had it." It was funny.

> And it was kind of interesting. I thought about the fact that I had a heart attack, and it seemed almost impossible. It was like my brain didn't want to accept it.

Other informants distanced themselves from the experience by doubting the veracity of the diagnosis. If they were able to maintain the belief that the diagnosis of a heart attack was an error, then they could maintain control:

> They told me I had a heart attack, but they never really convinced me. It wasn't until a week later that I was really convinced.

> They said it took them a long time to stabilize me and get me into the intensive care. . . . My kids were all coming in and sitting, and I was saying, "What are you doing here? I'm not dying. There's nothing wrong with me."

Once the diagnosis of a heart attack was made, the informants were all transferred to cardiac care units. Despite denying the diagnosis and distancing themselves from the events, the informants allowed their admission to the hospital. Many of the informants described themselves as "objects" or "automatons" who were cared for by others. Rather than taking active roles, things were done to them. The informants believed the hospital staff encouraged this distancing by instructing them to rest and stay calm, and they thought the staff expected cooperation. One informant described this state as "limbo," neither engaged in the hospital world nor in the security of day-to-day life: "It's kind of funny. You're kind of in and out of it. You're kind of stupid, but you remember what you say and hear." For some of the informants the distancing they described was inevitably aided by the administration of morphine, a drug commonly given to heart attack victims.

The informants remained distanced from the reality of their diagnoses and the hospital environment from one to seven days. During this period, many of them actively attempted to "prove" that they were not seriously ill. This "proof" took the form of challenging the authority of the hospital staff and rules or denying or ignoring the severity of their illness. For example, some of the informants said they attempted to do tasks that were not permitted, such as emptying their basins of water following their baths. One informant reported "sneaking off" the ward and exploring the hospital. Humor was also a mechanism used by the informants to distance themselves from the reality of their heart attacks:

> So they're [the informant's children] watching [the cardiac monitor]. They think they're going to get me excited, and I'm going to drop dead or

something. So one day I looked up at it, and as I'm twisting to look up, I noticed it went all funny, and then I twisted a little more and it went really funny. . . . So next time [my children] came, I started wiggling around, and I said, "Hey, now watch that T.V." . . . The older one said, "You're going to kill yourself. You can't do that." I said, "Oh, yes I can. Watch this. Isn't it neat!" But you gotta have some fun or else you'd drop dead in there.

Some informants attempted to "break the rules" which were imposed upon them in the hospital. For example, they attempted to get out of bed when they had been instructed to remain in bed, or they refused to comply with the wishes of the hospital staff by neglecting to inform the staff when their chest pain reoccurred. By refusing to take the hospital experience seriously the informants were able to remain distanced from the responsibilities and concerns which were associated with a possibly life threatening illness.

Over time it became extremely difficult for the informants to remain distanced. Family members, staff, and the presence of medical equipment provided constant reminders that the heart attack had indeed occurred and the informants slowly faced the reality of their heart attack. Some informants required irrevocable proof that they had experienced a heart attack. Once this proof was provided they began to come to terms with their heart attacks:

I was never really convinced until the cardio nurse came in [a week later]. . . . I asked her, "How do you know it's a heart attack?" So she says, "This little blip tells me it's a heart attack." And at that point . . . I feel that I accepted that it was a heart attack.

Stage Two: Coming to Terms

A heart attack can easily undermine one's sense of control over one's body and one's life in general. Prior to regaining a sense of control, the individual struggles to come to terms with the event. *Coming to terms* involves an effort to understand the event: why it occurred, what impact it has had, and what significance it has for the future. By coming to terms with the heart attack the individual is able to regain a sense of control over the event and over his or her life. Although some aspects of control cannot be regained through this process, it does enhance the individual's sense of predictability.

There are four phases that an individual usually completes when coming to terms with a heart attack. First, the individual faces his or her mortality. Through this process, he or she comes to some resolution regarding the experience of having survived a life threatening situation. Second, the individual makes sense out of what has occurred. To understand why the heart attack occurred gives the individual a sense of control over his or her destiny. Third, the individual faces the possible limitations that might occur as a result of the heart attack. They face the temporary loss of independence and grieve the losses they have experienced, both real and imagined. In turn, the culmination of these three phases contributes to the manner in which the fourth phase, the individual's attempts to develop an attitude toward the future, is managed. The attitude that the heart attack victim develops toward the future has a significant effect on the strategies that he or she will use in the subsequent stages of the adjustment process.

Facing One's Mortality

A heart attack is a potentially life threatening event, and individuals who experience a heart attack are faced with the possibility that they may not survive. Many of the individuals in this study had not contemplated the possibility of their death prior to the time of their heart attack. The ability to survive a life threatening event was considered a profound experience, and this event affected the way in which the informants envisioned their futures.

Initially, the thought of dying was extremely frightening for some informants:

I think I was scared. I thought, "Well, a heart attack, maybe it's the end."

Things go through your mind, you know: "Have I got long to live, or will my life be that much shorter?" And yet, I look around, and I think, "You know, I've had a good life."

As the informants contemplated the possibility of death they were often prompted to review their lives. They described two outcomes of their life review. First, some informants expressed a sense of being grateful for surviving. These individuals were generally optimistic about their futures. Other informants were less optimistic about the future and these individuals were unable to rid themselves of their preoccupation with death.

Those informants who were grateful for being given a "second chance to live" believed that having survived the heart attack was something to be thankful for:

> And on the fourth day, somebody gave me a newspaper . . . and as I read the obituary notices, I thought, "Oh my gosh, my name isn't there." And I knew I'd made it, and I sort of looked at the date, and I thought, "This is the day I'd be buried." And I felt very, very grateful.

This second chance allowed these informants the opportunity to cherish life, and many of them believed that they had not been living life to its fullest:

> I think life has taken on a different meaning in a lot of ways. Like, oh, even wanting to spend more time with my family, doing more for them, spending a little more time and doing things with them, taking them out and doing things with them.

This potent desire to live, however, was often dampened by the reality of the hospital setting and the limitations imposed by the heart attack. The informants were unable to "live life to its fullest" because they were weak, hospitalized, and dependent on others for support. Despite the restrictions they encountered, those informants who were able to maintain the belief that they had indeed been given a second chance were able to maintain a positive attitude about the future.

For other informants the threat of death was a profoundly negative experience. These individuals did not believe that the threat of death subsided with their symptoms. Rather than believe that they could make a "new start," they thought they might die an early death. For these informants the future was tentative:

> I said to my kids, "Don't get excited. Maybe I'll get better. Maybe I'll drop dead in a month. Who knows? There's no guarantee."

For these individuals their "brush with death" continued to be a frightening reminder of their mortality throughout the adjustment process. Accordingly, these informants were more cautious and pessimistic throughout the subsequent stages of the adjustment process.

The informants' beliefs regarding their mortality and futures were subject to change over time. The experiences that the informants had throughout the adjustment process affected the ways in which they *came to terms* with their heart attacks, and they often returned to the process of facing their mortality if they experienced serious symptoms in the course of their recovery or if they experienced an unexpectedly high degree of improvement.

Making Sense

Once the shock of the initial experience passes, the heart attack victim attempts to make sense of what has happened to him or her. Causal explanations of some kind were sought by each informant in this study. These explanations provided the victims with a sense of control. Finding a "reason" for the heart attack enabled these individuals to make sense of the event. Initially the heart attack made life seem unpredictable, but over time the informants were able to fit the reality of a heart condition into their lives:

> I spent a lot of time figuring out exactly what caused my heart attack. This was important because it allowed me to figure out exactly what could be done about it. . . . I'm 43 years old. Having had a heart attack, I don't want to put myself in these kinds of situations anymore.

The identification of the cause of the heart attack also provided the individual with a sense that his or her heart condition was a manageable problem. Many of the informants believed that knowing the "cause" provided the "key" to the cure. Those individuals who were unable to successfully determine the cause of their heart attacks had a great deal of difficulty managing their rehabilitation.

In order to make sense of the experience the informants reviewed their past lives in light of their present situations. Factors that were not considered important until the heart attack occurred were carefully scrutinized. Aspects of their lives, such as previous eating habits, took on new meaning. Most of the informants adjusted their perceptions of the past in order to make sense of the present:

See, I looked at myself, and I thought, "Well, I'm not overweight. I don't believe that I have high blood pressure. There's no stress that I can think of in the home environment. So it must be work related."

The combination of the high cholesterol level and the stress probably prompted it. So that's what I have to learn to avoid.

I was not truly a candidate for a heart attack because I eat a good diet and my weight is okay. Stress is really what caused it. I mean, there was just nothing I could do about it. I mean, that stress was just there.

Some individuals had difficulty identifying the cause of their heart attack. Despite careful consideration they were unable to make sense of the heart attack. These individuals ruminated about the cause of their heart attack until an explanation was found:

I kept thinking about it for about the first month after I got home . . . just going over in my mind "Why did this have to happen?" And then I'd sit and ponder over it.

Rather than identify the cause of their heart attacks, some individuals could only identify reasons why they should not have had a heart attack. These individuals viewed the heart attack as a threat that could not be explained. They later had difficulty making—and committing themselves to—any life-style changes as they were unable to identify a relationship between their previous life-styles and the occurrence of their heart attacks. These individuals believed that they had done everything possible to ward off the threat of heart disease, and they felt that somehow they had been betrayed:

I felt mad because I did all the right things. I thought, "I walk up and down eight flights. I swam every day. I walk wherever I can." I'd been doing all the right things. I'd also been watching my diet like mad. . . . I've always been interested in nutrition.

I felt that I shouldn't have had the heart attack, and yet I know it's hereditary in our family. But I don't smoke. . . . I've been eating pretty regular diets, and I don't drink that much. I've been pretty active. . . . I shouldn't get a heart attack. I'm too young. I don't smoke, and I'm pretty healthy.

All of the informants considered heart disease a life-style disease; consequently the process of seeking causal explanations was often associated with a sense of guilt. It was generally believed that heart attacks occur because individuals do "something wrong." Some informants went so far as to state that they *deserved* a heart attack because of the way they lived:

> It's the old story I guess. . . . I've worked, I've put in long hours, lots of worry, frustration, lots of stress. I've worked for this heart attack, and I got it. I mean it's mine. I've worked for this, and I guess you could say I got what I deserved.

Many of the informants felt a sense of remorse as they reviewed their lives. Some of them regretted the way they had lived their lives, while others wished they could "redo" parts of their lives: "Everyone goes through the things that you wish you could have done differently. The second time you'd do it differently, like the mistakes you've made."

The sense that the individual is personally responsible for his or her disease weighed heavily on many of the informants. This burden was felt because coronary artery disease was clearly considered a disease that can be avoided. For this reason, a heart condition was considered to be different from other diseases:

> I don't know how a person can opt out of not taking responsibility. And more so for a heart attack than cancer. I wouldn't feel the same way if I had cancer. I would say, "Hey, why me?" Or if I had been hit by a car, I could say, "Why me?" But I can't honestly say "Why me?" with a heart attack. I guess one could almost say I had it coming to me.

Some informants had been warned by friends and family members to change their life-styles prior to their heart attacks. These warnings were remembered by the informants and provided them with evidence of their responsibility: "In a way, I consider I've brought part of this problem onto myself. I certainly had enough warnings from the family. It was certainly talked about, and I didn't listen."

The process of making sense of the event was aided by health professionals who worked with these informants. The identification of risk factors is an integral part of the health history assessment conducted by physicians and nurses. As a result of these assessments many of the informants felt a cause for the heart attack was being sought by the health professionals. Often the questions asked by health professionals gave the informants clues as to what might have caused their heart attacks. This was considered helpful by some individuals because it provided them with a structure for examining causal explanations; however, some of the informants found the scrutiny of the health professionals distressing:

> There is a lot of finger pointing. You go along with them. And you start to think, "Something I did must have been wrong." 'Cause you're told this immediately. They tell you, "Well, let's see what you did that was wrong. Why did you get a heart attack?"

The informants attempted to make sense of the heart attack for their own benefit as well as for the benefit of others. The shock that family members and friends experienced when they learned of the diagnosis was often conveyed to the informants. Many informants believed that they needed to explain the cause of the heart attack to others. As stated earlier, many of the female informants believed that a heart attack is an illness that concerns only men; consequently, many of them were afraid that others would think they had done something "wrong." They felt ashamed of having had a heart attack and the insinuations that they encountered were at times devastating:

> I've said that I could have thought of many things that could happen to me, but I never, ever in my life gave thought to a heart attack because I couldn't. . . . My friends and my neighbors, I don't think there's one of them that hasn't said, "How come *you* got a heart attack?"

> You know, everybody thinks about it once: "How come you're having a heart attack? You're too young, you're too skinny, you don't eat fat, you don't eat salt." It's like you had to have done something bad to have a heart attack.

Making sense of a heart attack can be difficult for some individuals because of its hidden nature. The heart attack is not a condition one can visualize; consequently, once the pain had subsided some of the informants in this study were left feeling that it was all over. These individuals had difficulty believing that the heart attack was "real": "I was alive. It didn't seem anything could happen to me after it was over." Although symptoms of fatigue and occasional pain persisted they did not provide the informants with visible reminders of the heart attack:

> Now if I was laying there with an artery pumping blood, I'd be scared. . . . That's a visible thing you can see. You know you've had the cookie then. But with a heart attack, the pain goes away after they give you a shot.

> If you got a broken leg, you got it in a cast. You can see that, and that's a daily reminder. But here you are with a heart attack that you cannot see, and you're looking at your body and thinking, "I'm okay, I look okay."

Until these informants encountered their limitations they had difficulty believing the heart attack would have a permanent effect on their lives. If they encountered difficulties in the months following the initial heart attack the informants often returned to the strategy of trying to make sense of the heart attack. Sometimes causal explanations were disregarded because the informants found that the explanations they had developed were not credible, and in these situations the individuals returned to the strategy of attempting to make sense of the situation.

Facing Limitations

An essential aspect of coming to terms with one's heart attack is facing the resultant limitations. A heart attack can have a huge impact on an individual's life, so before coming to terms with the heart attack one must consider the implications the heart attack holds for the future, the obstacles that might lie ahead, and the plans that must be altered. Many of the limitations that an individual initially considers will not actually exist in the future; nevertheless, these perceived limitations have a strong impact on how the individual comes to terms with the heart attack. For example, if the limitations are perceived to be insurmountable the individual will have difficulty regaining a sense of control over his or her life.

The informants in this study were faced with limitations that were imposed on them by the hospital staff from the moment they entered the hospital system. Most of their activities were restricted including walking, shaving, eating, and visiting. These limitations served as strong reminders to the informants that they were not well:

I realized they weren't letting me out of bed. I couldn't even swing my feet over to the side of the bed. I was on a liquid diet . . . and then they told me I had a really bad one. Oh well, I guess I did.

As the informants' health improved they were gradually allowed to increase their levels of activity. At this point most informants experienced the physical limitations that were imposed on them as a result of the heart attack. While lying in bed most of the informants were unaware of their inabilities; however, by the third or fourth day of hospitalization they began to take short walks and they became aware of their physical limitations. Most of them described sensations of fatigue and weakness. Simple tasks such as bathing and walking proved exhausting:

They told me a lot of things I couldn't do right away . . . and that kind of made me think, "Well gee, am I that sick?" . . . But the minute I tried doing something, then I realized they knew what they were talking about. . . . The first time they walked me down the hall I was just exhausted, and I thought, "Well gee, does a heart attack take that much out of you?"

Faced with devastating physical limitations many informants pondered their future. They feared that they would never regain their strength: "I thought, 'Boy if this is the way you are going to be all your life, this is rotten.' And that's when I started getting disappointed." By far the greatest fear for these individuals was that they would remain permanently disabled: "Initially, I believed that I was going to be a semi-invalid for the rest of my life. . . . I was pretty depressed."

Many of the informants feared that the limitations they faced would be permanent. A sense that an irrevocable change had occurred prompted many of them to grieve the loss of a previously enjoyed life-style. Many informants spent time considering all of the activities they would no longer be able to do. These considerations were based on their current inabilities rather than on an understanding of how they might improve: "I thought, 'Oh, will I have to quit my bowling and my golfing? Do I have to quit all of the things I enjoy? My life is going to get so boring.' "

Although all of the informants were told they would improve, many feared that they would experience permanent disability of some kind. In order to cope with these fears they engaged in *anticipatory worrying*. *Anticipatory worrying* involved ruminating about the worst possible outcomes of the heart attack. Many informants believed that if one prepared for the worst, the future could be faced. For example, one informant decided that he would never be able to drive again because he believed he was unable to change a tire. This type of belief was not unusual as the heart attack had this effect on many of the informants.

The informants said that they worried for three days to two weeks about their potential limitations. Most of them were able to grieve their potential losses and subsequently place their losses behind them. They recognized that they had to begin to make some adjustments. In order to make this transition they constructed an understanding of the heart attack that would allow them to continue with the adjustment process and end the grieving period. They developed an attitude toward the future which, in turn, provided them with a sense of direction.

Looking to the Future

Having faced their mortality and the limitations that the heart attack imposed and having attempted to make sense out of what occurred, the informants believed that they were faced with two options: They could continue to ruminate about what happened to them or they could look to the future and attempt to make adjustments. The speed with which the informants attempted to look to the future varied. Although some informants were able to move quickly to this final phase of coming to terms with their heart condition, others had difficulty resolving their feelings about their mortality or their potential limitations. The way in which an informant envisioned his or her future was significant as it was this factor which had the greatest impact on the selection of subsequent strategies in the adjustment process.

One informant described an "attitude" as "the position you are going to take towards the attack." The majority of the informants believed that a "positive attitude" made the greatest contribution to the adjustment process. It was believed that if one were positive "you could lick it, instead of it licking you." Not every informant, however, was initially able to develop a positive attitude. The attitudes that the informants initially displayed can be divided into two groups: those with a positive attitude and those with an attitude that one must "wait and see" what the future would hold (see Figure 2.3).

The informants said a positive attitude involved a belief that they would improve, that they would be able to adjust successfully. In turn, this belief aided the informants in developing a sense of control. For these informants the future seemed manageable and they felt that the obstacles to adjustment were not insurmountable. Although the informants wanted to possess a positive attitude, many found that they had to spend time convincing themselves that they would recuperate:

> I think I'm looking forward to a good life, you know? I'm sure everything is going to be good for me. I just have to look at things positively and think, "If I look after myself, I'm going to have a good life. Maybe this was just a little warning. Maybe if I look after myself, I'm going to have a good life with my grandchildren."

The way in which an individual makes sense of the heart attack appears to have a significant impact on his or her attitude. For example, informants who were able to "pinpoint" the reason for their heart attacks developed specific ideas about how they could improve their health, and they viewed the heart attack as a "warning." They believed that if they rectified "the problem" they would live long and healthy lives:

> So it's happened, and I guess I have to resign myself that it is a warning, and it was a very fortunate warning because within the next two weeks of my heart attack two of our friends didn't have that second chance. It was one heart attack, and they no longer exist type of thing. So in one way, I guess, I take it as a warning, and I have to adapt to the fact that it is a warning and start to pace myself.

One informant said she was "grateful" for her heart attack because it forced her to make necessary changes in her life. Individuals such as this informant were generally keen to make life-style changes. They enthusiastically incorporated the changes suggested to them by health professionals, particularly if they believed that the changes would resolve the problems which they believed had caused their

Positive Attitude	*"Wait and See"*
Confidence in recovery	Fear of being permanently disabled
"Knowing" the cause(s)	Inability to understand "why"
	Anger - "I did everything right"
"Gratefulness" for a second chance	Knowledge of why they "shouldn't have had a heart attack"
	Fear of the possibility of death
Possession of specific plans for rehabilitation.	Uncertainty regarding the future
	Reluctance to commit to plans
Perceptions that limitations are manageable	Perceptions that limitations are insurmountable

Figure 2.3. Factors that Affect Attitudes Regarding the Future

heart attacks. These individuals were less amenable to changes that, in their minds, had no bearing on the problem.

Some of the individuals who were unable to pinpoint causes for their heart attacks were still able to develop positive attitudes. Many of these informants decided to adopt this attitude simply because they wanted to live: "It's not time to roll over and play dead yet." Other informants simply refused to believe that life was over. For a few this urge to live was sparked by the realization that they had been given a second chance. By facing their mortality they had developed a new appreciation for life. One informant described his heart attack as "the best thing that could have happened to [him]." When asked why, he said, "I'll be a better person for what has happened."

The informants who remained angry or depressed and unable to make sense of their heart attacks had great difficulty considering the future. Although many of these individuals desired a positive outlook, they believed they had nothing about which to be positive.

These individuals continued to view life as tentative. They doubted that their health would improve. They were frightened of what the future held for them. These individuals said they had great difficulty deciding how they would deal with the future: "I've just got to wait and see how good I'm going to get." Those individuals who felt they had to wait and see were tentative about specific plans: "If I knew what caused it, I wouldn't do it again. I just don't know what caused it, so I don't know how to fix it." These individuals believed that they could not be positive about the future until they resolved the uncertainties that they associated with their heart condition.

The way in which an informant envisioned his or her future changed throughout the course of the adjustment process: "You tend to follow the direction you are looking toward. If you feel bad, you won't do well. If you feel good, like you are going to get better, then you will." As improvements were experienced and uncertainty dissipated, those informants who felt that life was tentative were able to anticipate the future with a greater sense of confidence. On the other hand, one informant who initially held a strong belief that she would improve faced many complications during the adjustment process. As a result of these difficulties she was unable to maintain a positive attitude. She became cynical about her future. She was unwilling to make plans and she believed that nothing she did would help her to improve.

Stage Three: Learning to Live

A heart attack disrupts one's sense of control to such a degree that one must learn, once again, how to live. In order to learn how to live the heart attack victim must negotiate through an adjustment process that is plagued with uncertainties and doubts. These individuals must discover a way to put their lives back together. They must learn to trust their bodies again and construct a life-style that they can tolerate and maintain. This stage includes three phases:

- preserving a sense of self,
- minimizing the uncertainty, and
- establishing guidelines for living.

There is a reciprocal relationship between the second and third stages of the adjustment process. The ability of the individual to come to terms with the event affects the strategies used in the third stage, and in turn the strategies used in the third stage affect the process of coming to terms with the event (see Figure 2.4). For example, if the informants found that the strategies they selected were ineffective they would return to the process of coming to terms. Similarly, those individuals who feared that they would remain physically disabled returned to the process of coming to terms once they experienced some improvement. The attitudes that a heart attack victim holds are subject to change over time; consequently, the processes of coming to terms with the event and learning to live are cyclical.

Preserving Self

A heart attack disrupts one's sense of self in that it undermines self-confidence and self-worth. A heart attack threatens one's independence, and consequently, there is a dramatic shift in one's roles and responsibilities. Throughout these changes, the heart attack victim must struggle to preserve a sense of self. He or she must struggle to maintain a personal identity other than one of *patient* or *invalid*. This was one of the most taxing struggles for many of the informants in this study:

> You've got to prove to yourself that you are not a cripple because to be a cripple is to be a loser. Isn't it? You know from the minute you start kindergarten you're taught not to be a loser. The only thing that counts in our society is to be a winner. Losers are nothing.

The informants indicated that much of their sense of self-worth was related to what they did as mothers, fathers, workers, spouses, men, and women. The heart attack disrupted these well-defined roles. To have these roles stripped away was often devastating: "I think the most difficult thing was feeling useless. You couldn't do anything." To be considered incapable, by one's self and by others, was extremely threatening: "I just don't like somebody doing everything for me and thinking I am really restricted."

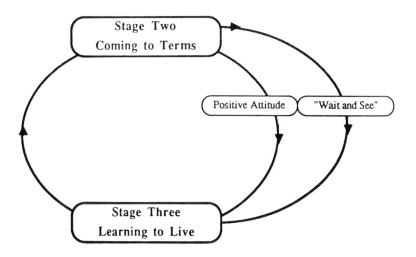

Figure 2.4. The Reciprocal Relationship Between the Second and Third Stages of the Adjustment Process

All of the informants said they were anxious to return to their previous life-styles. Some of them indicated that they were "raring to go" before they were discharged from the hospital. Others wanted to return to their previous life-styles; however, they were afraid that they would experience a second heart attack if they pushed themselves too hard. Despite these desires the informants were unable to "pick up where they left off." All of the informants initially complained of extreme fatigue. In addition they were all informed by various health care professionals that many of their usual activities had to be curtailed for a period of six weeks to three months. Most informants were given instructions regarding what they should not do. Because of these restrictions and their physical limitations they were unable to resume, as one informant said, "a full life." In order to preserve a sense of self under these restrictive conditions, the informants used two strategies: First, they managed their role transitions, and second, they attempted to balance their needs and supports.

Managing Role Transitions

The individual who experiences a heart attack is quickly and without warning cast into the role of patient. Many of the informants said they were extremely uncomfortable with the patient role: "I'm not used to being waited on. I didn't like to be waited on. I wanted to do my own thing." Both the men and women in this study had difficulty accepting the patient role; however, the reasons for this difficulty were different for the male and female informants. Many of the female informants said they preferred to give rather than receive care: "I like to do things for other people, but I've never really wanted to be waited on." The female informants in this study tended to see themselves as caregivers not care receivers.

Many of the women in this study attempted to protect their mothering roles. They felt particularly uncomfortable when their children attempted to provide comfort. In order to maintain their mothering roles, the women demonstrated care and concern for their family members by minimizing their own conditions:

> I didn't want them to get too upset because it was a bad time for them, too. . . . So I would just try to minimize everything to them. I'd say things like "Don't you know it'll be okay." I felt I had to be cheerful, otherwise they would have just gone overboard.

Other women discouraged their family members from visiting them in the hospital in order not to burden their loved ones. Many of the female informants said they spent a great deal of their time in the hospital worrying about how their husbands and children would handle their illness. One woman said that "it was harder on the children than it was on [me]."

The majority of male informants enjoyed the attention of family members while hospitalized: "I liked the attention. It made me feel loved. I mean, it's the clearest signal I've had in our 16 years of marriage that she really loves me." Rather than discourage the attention of family members, most of the male informants encouraged it.

The major aspect of the patient role that the male informants disliked was the threat to their breadwinning role. Many of the men were concerned about being absent from work and some of them attempted to have their work brought to them in the hospital:

I was always doing something and then, all of the sudden, to do nothing. I found it very frustrating in the hospital to sit and do nothing. I felt that if someone brought me some work to do, I could do it, and they could pick it up and take it back. But no, they wouldn't let me do that either because that's what put me in there.

Being a patient prevented the male informants from continuing their breadwinner role, and without this role, they felt "useless" : "You are the breadwinner of the family. You have the status. And all of the sudden, you go from having the status to being nothing." The female informants who were employed outside of their homes were not initially concerned with the continuation of their work. Their initial concerns focused on the care of their family members.

The majority of the informants were eager to leave the hospital; however, two informants said they felt comfortable in the patient role and were anxious about their discharge: "The hospital staff know exactly what's happening. . . . I felt safe and secure while I was in the hospital." These particular individuals were extremely hesitant about the future and required much reassurance. Neither of them had come to terms with the heart attack prior to discharge from the hospital:

I was afraid to leave. I thought, you know, "What if I have another heart attack?" At the hospital, I'd be attended to right away. . . . I mean, they bring you your pills at a certain time, and you're looked after pretty good. And then you think, "Gee, when you go home, you're on your own. Am I going to make it? Am I going to manage?" Yes, it was a worry. Oh, the first week I think I was so scared at home. I was scared of having another heart attack and not getting to the hospital in time.

Once the informants were discharged from the hospital they were faced with the challenge of assuming their previous roles. The informants were told by health care professionals that their full rehabilitation would require six weeks to six months. Many of the informants were discouraged by the length of this rehabilitation period. The thought of "taking it easy" for three months seemed interminable to many; in fact all of the informants said they felt useless. Many of the informants felt caught between the roles they had once enjoyed and the patient role. They did not feel "legitimately sick," yet they did not feel well enough to resume their previous roles: "To be just not able to do anything, just to be lying around and being useless, I think this was the most difficult thing out of the whole heart attack." Several factors impeded the informants from resuming their previous roles: the efforts of their family members to protect them, the restrictions that health care professionals placed on them, and their physical limitations.

Many informants believed that being restricted from certain tasks diminished the value of their existence. They felt that who they were as people was directly related to what they could accomplish. To have their abilities limited by a heart attack was devastating. The informants found it difficult to fill their time at home, and the meaning that life once held for them was diminished:

> I find the worst part about it is sitting at home being idle. It is very frustrating. I guess I was a workaholic to a point. And to sit and not do anything, well. Like, when I was discharged I said, "Well, now I can go home. I can do some exercises." I was overweight. I knew that without having been told. I could do some exercises to strengthen, and as soon as I talked to my doctor, he says, "You don't do anything." I says, "Well, can't I?" He says, "You can go and you can walk, but you're not to leave the house." For the first week, I was housebound. I couldn't go anywhere. . . . I found it very frustrating to get up and not have a purpose in life except to maybe exist until the next day.

All of the informants believed that their relationships with their family members had changed as a result of their heart attacks. The return home was often awkward as their family members treated them "differently." This change in behavior on the part of family members reinforced the fact that the informants had changed. Many of them said they felt extremely uncomfortable with their family members' attempts to protect them: "Instead of me doing everything, there was everybody doing everything for me. That seemed really strange because I always take care of my own household." Most informants said they allowed their family members to care for them for the first three to seven days. After this period of time being treated as invalids became intolerable. They felt they could no longer acquiesce to their families' demands to protect them and they attempted to assert their independence.

All but one of the informants described a situation in which they had to assert themselves as a person and reestablish a role for themselves in the family. They were unable to tolerate the protectiveness of their family members as this protectiveness made them feel like "invalid[s] who [were] unable to think and feel for [themselves]." They believed that they had to let their family members know that they were capable adults:

> Well, there was a little anger building up in me because she's the oldest one, and she was the most protective. Like, I would get up out of my chair, and "No, no mom, don't. Where are you going? What are you going to do?" "I want to go to the bathroom." "Well, okay." And if I'd get up to do something." No, no mom, no, no. You can't do that. No, no. Let me do it. Don't go upstairs again, oh no." And she'd be walking behind me and follow me up the stairs. I said, "I can go up and down the stairs twice a day, and that's all I do." I'd go to take a spoon out of the cupboard drawer, "No, no mom, sit down. I'll do that for you." Well, it just finally got to me. . . . So I finally just had to yell at her. And I yelled at her really good.

Attempts to assert themselves were often difficult for the informants to manage as they appreciated the care and attention offered to them by their families. Indeed most of the informants recognized that they required some support, yet they wanted to believe that they were "independent and in control." But the informants knew that by asserting their independence they ran the risk of shutting the door to all assistance.

Many of the informants said their family members believed they were less capable as a result of their heart attacks. For example, two of the women in this study described being offended because their daughters no longer asked them to care for their grandchildren. Family members often did everything possible to shield the informants from possible stress. According to one informant, the reason for this highly protectionist attitude was due to the fact that "they don't want to think that they're going to be the cause of something else happening to you." The result of this treatment was a feeling of isolation and of not being needed. This isolation was stressful for the informants. For example, one informant told her children, "You're going to make me have another heart attack if you don't let me do anything."

It was often difficult to relinquish the tasks that an informant associated with his or her particular role. To allow others to perform these tasks was often frustrating:

> I used to enjoy going out and shoveling snow if I had the time. It was a period of tranquility where I was out there on my own. I could think what I wanted to think. I solved a lot of problems at work, just a general feeling that you could do what you wanted to do, and you didn't have to think. I really enjoyed that period. And now, [my wife] has to do the shoveling. [It] was . . . frustrating [that] she had to do the shoveling.

The realization that certain tasks were prohibited was difficult for the informants as it reinforced their feelings of being useless: "You just can't sit for the rest of your life without doing anything." These restrictions also affected the ways in which the informants perceived themselves. One informant was asked by a stranger to help lift a package shortly after returning home. Although he was tempted to agree, he knew he should not assist as the package was extremely heavy: "I thought she was going to say, 'Big strong man like you, you should be able to pick it up.' But she didn't."

Although most of the informants were reluctant to discuss the resumption of sexual activity, one informant indicated that although he was aware that he was able to resume sexual activity he was afraid that others might believe he was impotent:

> I'm sitting there listening. Probably it's a misconception that people with heart attacks can't have sex, and they asked me at this meeting if I was coming back to work. And I said, "Yes," and they said, "Why?" I said, "Well, there's no girls at home that want to play games." And they turned around, and they said, "Hey, you watch it. You have had a heart attack. You can't have sex." And I said, "Where in the hell did you get an idea like that?" It's not me that needs to learn about the sex. It's the others who don't have the heart attack.

For this informant, the heart attack threatened his role as a sexual human being. The actual resumption of sexual activity was not as important as the beliefs that others held regarding his sexual capabilities. In order to cope with this threat he believed that he had to "set the record straight."

Many of the informants found it difficult to say "no" to certain activities and tasks. The heart attack left them with no visible limitations, and unless they were told acquaintances had no knowledge that the informants had experienced a heart attack. This often caused a dilemma. To "tell" was to admit one was not well and this created the risk of being considered an invalid. To avoid telling was to run the risk of being asked or expected to perform activities beyond one's abilities. One woman attempted to resolve this problem by refusing to wear her makeup once she returned home. She believed that without her makeup she would look tired and would not have to deal with the issue of whether to "tell." Another informant said he used the following approach when faced with the question of whether to inform others that he had experienced a heart attack:

> I find that if you tell them outright then they're not playing games. But if they don't ask me, I'm not going to turn around and tell them. A guy asked me to help shove his car, push his car over. And I said, "I can't do that." He looked at me, and he says, "You should be able to put a lot of weight behind it." I said, "Look, I've had a heart attack. I'm not going to shove your car." He looked at me, and I said, "But if you want, I'll push it, provided you accept all the problems."

Many of the informants felt caught between the patient role and their previous roles. They were not well enough to carry on as before, yet they were not sick enough to remain a patient. Although this transitional state became easier to manage as time progressed, the informants used a number of strategies to manage their role transitions. When necessary, they emphatically asserted their independence. In situations where they were unable to be independent they either learned to incorporate their limitations into their life style or they began to bend the rules. Learning to incorporate these limitations was no easy task:

> You have to adapt to the fact that you cannot do what you used to do, and it's a blow to your ego because you want to try and do things. . . . When you find that you better not, for your own good, believe me, your ego takes a plunge. You know you have to learn that you can't do certain things, and that's all there is to it.

All of the limitations experienced by the informants left them feeling dependent and useless.

In this study it was found that the women bent the rules more than the men. Although many men were anxious to return to work, their employers' regulations and physicians' advice held them back. Although most of the men in this study returned to work within a three month period following their heart attack, most of the women resumed all of their household responsibilities within six to eight weeks.

Rather than remain dependent on others, many of the women in this study chose to bend the rules regarding housework. They found it extremely difficult to return to their homes, to "their places of work," and not resume the necessary tasks: "I felt I wanted to do my own housework and do my own thing and do what I wanted. And I found it hard not doing what I wanted." The women in this study strongly believed that no one could do their housework as well as they could, and in particular they considered their husbands incapable of "see[ing] the corners" that needed cleaning: "I think if it wasn't for the woman, I think a lot of things would slide. If we expected men to do certain things, they wouldn't get done." These informants felt it was intolerable to do nothing when the house was not clean:

> Well, I'm sort of a bit of a clean-freak, and if I see things, anything that needs to be done, I'll just do it, you know. If I see just anything, a little bit of dust there, or here, or whatever, I'd have to get my duster.

Some of the women initially allowed their children and husbands to help them; however, this did not prove satisfactory for long. The resumption of housework was "an automatic thing." Some of the women realized that they were resuming activities at a quicker pace than was recommended by health care professionals, however, they saw no alternative. Many of them felt that they could not ask their husbands to iron the clothes, make the beds, and prepare the meals. Most of them were able to enlist the help of their husbands with the vacuuming and floor washing; however, by the end of the first six weeks they did not feel comfortable requesting this assistance. Many of the women in this study did not view housework as "work." They did not believe that exertion was required for tasks such as tidying and ironing:

> One day I started getting the angina. I mentioned it to them at the clinic. I had done, you know, the beds and tidied the bathrooms, and then in the

afternoon, I went down, and I ironed, and they said, "Well you know, you should iron maybe two pieces at a time to begin with." And here I stood there for half an hour. But I was so mad at myself. I kept on saying, "I'm sure I can do half an hour's ironing. I'm not doing anything."

Some of the women felt pressured by health care professionals to ask their husbands to assist them with the household tasks; however, these women felt it was not fair to ask their husbands for assistance with "women's work":

It's a different world now with both parents working. With my children, both parents are working, and I feel that the husband should help. But when I had my children, my husband worked shift work twelve hours a day, and you didn't expect him to come home and do the dishes and stuff like that. It's pretty hard. It's hard to change him now, you know. And I don't intend to make him change. I mean I don't.

Many of the men in this study said they helped with housework while they were recuperating in order to "fill in time." They did not resume the same amount of activity as quickly as the women in this study, however. Additionally, those women who worked outside of their homes deemed it necessary to resume household activities long before they returned to their paid employment.

Acting against his physician's advice one man in this study returned to work three weeks following his heart attack. His decision to return to work was based on the belief that he was "useless sitting around doing nothing," and he was unable to tolerate the absence of any useful activity:

I'm not a jock. I have no use for exercise. It's a nonproductive kind of activity for me. I like to say at the end of the day, "Well, I've accomplished this." But you step off those exercise machines and what have you accomplished? Nothing.

Although most of the informants could accept a short period of "time out" from their regular routine, knowing that a period of recuperation would benefit their health, this man was unable to remain at home and continue to feel valued as a person. He was never convinced that he could do anything to improve his health. He believed that the heart attack was an inevitability that had to be accepted and forgotten. He believed that the only option open to him was to return to work. By immersing himself in his work he was able to return to a role in which he felt comfortable. In the first months back at work he would remain at work for the entire day and returned home exhausted. He would retire for the evening immediately on his return home and would remain in bed until the next day. Remaining at work was so important to this man that he virtually ceased to function in any other role. He isolated himself from family members and friends. He was willing to make this sacrifice in order to continue working: "I've sacrificed my leisure time for my work, and that was my choice. . . . So again, I guess my life is still regimented and revolves around work."

This informant's behavior clearly exemplifies the importance of roles to one's integrity. He was extremely threatened by the potential loss of his role as a worker. He had witnessed many of his friends develop health problems and then "vegetate." He felt that "if you're capable of doing the work, [then] a paycheck for not doing it [is] a bit of welfare." Although this informant was a blatant example, many of the informants in this study struggled in similar ways to reclaim their roles. The reclaiming of these roles was extremely important to the informants as the resumption of previously held roles provided a strong indication of improvement in their health. On the other hand, the failure to resume roles provided proof that they were ill.

Balancing Needs and Supports

Initially, the individual who has experienced a heart attack is faced with a loss of control. He or she is uncertain about the future and is unable to function independently. In order to regain a sense of control the individual requires the assistance of others. Closely related to the strategy of managing role transitions is the strategy of balancing needs and supports. Once he or she returns home the individual who experienced a heart attack is often overwhelmed by the assistance offered by others. In order to preserve a sense of self-worth, individuals must attempt to balance their needs with available supports. An integral part of balancing needs and supports is the ability to request and refuse assistance.

Four outcomes are possible as a result of the individual's attempt to balance his or her perceived needs with supports (see Figure 2.5). The individuals who believe they need a great deal of support and who have the supports available to meet those needs are depicted

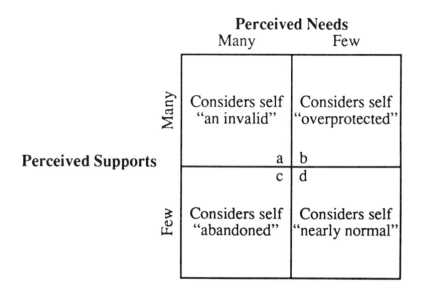

Figure 2.5. Balancing Needs and Supports

in Cell *a* of Figure 2.5. Although most of the informants believed they belonged to this category during the initial stages of hospitalization, many of them found it difficult to remain in this situation. To be constantly receiving assistance for a protracted period of time left the informants feeling incapable and indebted to others. If the informants believed that they needed a great deal of support and this support was provided unconditionally, their beliefs about being unable to care for themselves were reinforced. They began to feel like invalids, unable to care for themselves and dependent on others. Constantly requiring and accepting support intensified their feelings of uselessness:

> Well, [it is] a real useless feeling. Here I haven't got the energy to do this or do that or accomplish something, and this is real upsetting. . . . I think everybody needs to be useful. If you have a feeling of being useless, I think you feel what's the use of living sort of thing. So you need to feel useful.

In particular, many of the informants had difficulty accepting the unconditional support of their families. Whereas the support provided by health care providers could be rationalized on the basis that they were "doing their jobs," the support of family members reinforced the informants' feelings of disability:

> You eventually don't want to think that you are that bad, that things have to be disrupted. You want to feel that you're better maybe than what you are. . . . It's like the more they fuss over me, the more I'm going to feel like I'm really an invalid or something. Don't disrupt your lives, go about and do what you're doing with your families, and you know, I'll be okay.

In order to preserve a sense of self, individuals who believed that they required considerable support often attempted to demonstrate their love and care for their families. It was essential that they were able to reciprocate the care that they received as caring for others enabled them to preserve a sense that they were whole human beings. Reciprocity was an essential element in the balancing of needs and supports. If the informants believed they were incapable of reciprocating support, either immediately or in the future, they felt devalued as human beings.

As the informants began to improve and gain strength in the immediate weeks following their discharge, their need for support diminished. If their family members were not cognizant of their improvements and continued to provide support in the same ways, without modification, the informants felt overprotected (see Figure 2.5, Cell *b*). In this case, supports outweighed needs, a situation that was extremely difficult for the informants. Often they felt obliged to accept the offered support as they believed that to refuse the offered support might result in the end of all support: "I was wishing that they wouldn't fuss so much, but then on the other hand, if I told them not to fuss, I might be rejected or something." The acceptance of support that was not required left the informants feeling useless and indebted to their families. Many of the informants described themselves as "dolls" or "babies" who received care regardless of their needs or desires, and they considered the attitudes of friends and families condescending.

The ways varied in which informants coped with this imbalance of needs and supports. One individual found the protectiveness of his wife intolerable. He felt degraded by her constant attempts to protect him. He believed that "she was almost creating a cardiac cripple out of [him]." He felt she was attempting to control him in her efforts to protect him from the outside world. His solution to this imbalance of needs and supports was to leave his wife, and subsequently he divorced her.

Other informants were able to handle the overprotective behavior of their family members. These individuals felt their acceptance of support was a favor they were bestowing on their concerned family members. They believed the least they could do to show their appreciation was to let their family members express their concern:

> It doesn't bother me because I know in my mind, I know in my heart that it's not really needed as far as I'm concerned. But if it's going to make someone else feel more comfortable, by all means, because it doesn't hurt me at all.

Consequently, the balance of needs and supports was restored. By recognizing their family members' need to support them the informants were able to reciprocate the care and concern they initially received from their family. In fact by accepting support the informants believed that they were supporting their family members.

Some informants who were unable to accept the protectiveness of their families used a third approach to restore a balance between needs and supports: They refused to accept the offered support. As described earlier, this often involved the informants demanding that their families and friends allow them the space necessary to "learn their own limits." In order to make their point they used a variety of tactics. They screamed, explained, and discussed their point of view in order to let their family members know that they were intelligent adults who could use judgment and assume self-responsibility. One informant employed a rather unique approach to explain to her children that they no longer had to worry:

> I made a point of telling them "I pulled the fridge out today and scrubbed behind, and boy, it must have been six months. You should have seen the dust." Just to let them know I can do things, and it doesn't bother me at all. And now they know, they don't have to get excited.

There were two informants in this study who believed their needs exceeded the offered support (see Figure 2.5, Cell *c*). One of these individuals was divorced. She had few friends as she spent all her time working and caring for her family. Her teenage daughter who lived at home was not "able to provide" the care and support that she believed she required, and her strategy for dealing with this perceived lack of support was to "try [her] best to manage." Often she felt totally isolated and "abandoned." She eventually realized that she would have to seek new avenues of support if she was going to be able to continue a normal life. She described this period in time without support as "devastating." She relied on her own resources, particularly on her belief that she was going to improve: "I just kept looking forward to feeling better."

The other informant who believed that his needs for support were not met felt that his wife "resented the fact that [he] had the heart attack." He sensed that she was unable to respect his need to recuperate:

> There's resentment there because she gets up and goes to work in the morning, and I stay home sleeping. She feels there's nothing really wrong with me right now. Really, I don't think there's anything wrong with me right now.

The perception that his wife thought there was nothing wrong caused him to believe that he was malingering. Initially he tried to encourage his wife to read some literature about rehabilitation following heart attack, but she refused. He felt he was unable to convince her of his need for recuperation and he felt abandoned. He believed that she should have been able to express some form of concern. Eventually he responded to this lack of concern by pushing himself as hard as he could in order to prove his abilities and disprove the belief that he was ill or malingering. Rather than continue to ask for support he attempted to change his behavior in order to match her expectations.

An essential element in achieving a balance between needs and supports was a spirit of cooperation. The cooperative spirit involved the ability of the informant and his or her family members to freely give and receive support (see Figure 2.5, Cell *d*). These individuals described themselves as "nearly normal" in that they felt both respected and cared for as whole human beings. They felt neither dependent nor abandoned; rather, they felt capable of playing a role in their own adjustment. In this context needs were not viewed as separate from supports; rather, there was a mutual exchange of support between the informants and their family members. A spirit of cooperation existed which involved the family members respecting and trusting the abilities of the informant and the informant respecting the need of his or her family to express concern:

> It was just a case of helping each other a little bit, you know. It wasn't like he was perfectly healthy and he could have taken over and [done] things for me. . . . We managed together to get by. . . . We talk more. More conversation, more getting things out in the open.

When the informants and their families were able to cooperate, supporting and respecting each other's needs, the informants said they felt a sense of control. They felt encouraged and cared for, and as a result of their family members' encouragement and care they were able to develop a sense of trust in themselves. In turn, this enabled them "to venture out and find [their] own limits."

Minimizing Uncertainty

Individuals who experience heart attacks are faced with uncertainties regarding activity resumption, diet, and stress management. They are uncertain about "what to do and how to do it." In particular, when they return home and are removed from the hospital support system they have difficulty making decisions regarding their own care. They are aware that their bodies have changed and that the "rules of living" have been altered, yet they are uncertain about these new rules. In addition, individuals who are unsure about their abilities to recover are concerned about the possibility of death and are afraid they will not improve.

The informants in this study described a variety of uncertainties which they faced and attempted to minimize. Many of them were unsure about how quickly they would be able to recover, and the course of recovery seemed vague to many:

> If you're cut open to be operated on, you know that in time that's going to heal. You're going to feel better once your strength comes back. But with this. . . . I'd never had one before, so I was a bit leery about just how I was going to make out.

Thinking that I wouldn't be able to get back to the level I was before, you know, 'cause you don't know. It's an unknown fact. You just have to wait and see. Nobody can tell you because nobody knows. Everything is uncertain.

Many of the informants said they wanted to know in "black and white" what they could and could not do as they felt ill equipped to make decisions on their own:

It would be nice to know exactly why and when and how right down to the minute. And it would be nice if you knew all of this right at the very beginning . . . because it's the uncertainty that makes you feel so bad. You'd like to have some answers.

This uncertainty affected every aspect of the informants' lives. Not only were they unsure about what decisions to make, they remained uncertain about the decisions they had made:

I went to a hockey game, and while I was watching, I was getting so excited I had to actually take a few nitro pills because of my angina pain. I don't know if it was even advisable for me to go there because fellows have died of situations like that.

This uncertainty was also experienced in terms of their ability to engage in rehabilitation programs. They were unsure about what was expected of them and they were uncertain if they would be able to handle the exercise programs. Even the equipment presented uncertainties:

I was quite apprehensive about it, you know, because you have to learn to take your pulse and work on the machines and the treadmill and that. And I thought, "What if I can't manage?"

Many of the informants were uncertain because they felt vulnerable. They were afraid that they might inadvertently trigger another heart attack. These individuals felt as though their bodies had betrayed them; and because they had been betrayed once before they thought it could happen again:

> One reason I was pretty careful about what I did physically and why I wanted to be under observation was because I had no idea what in the world I might do to trigger this again.

In light of this uncertainty, every action was carefully scrutinized. Nothing could be done without considering the heart attack:

> There were a ton of uncertainties, mostly like "Can I lift this or not lift that? Can I spend four hours out?" Walking around, I mean, how much is too much? Which activity should I do, and which ones shouldn't I do?

For those individuals who persisted in the belief that they would not get better, the uncertainties of living were omnipresent. Two informants were afraid to sleep at night because they feared they might never wake up. Another informant confided that she was afraid that she might have another heart attack while in the bath. Her solution was to complete her bathing as quickly as possible. These uncertainties were paralyzing for some of the informants. For example, one informant refused to leave her home because she feared something untoward might happen to her.

Some of the informants said they were uncertain because they could not understand what had happened to their heart. For these individuals it was extremely important to understand the "functions" of the heart. To understand how the heart functioned provided these informants with an understanding of what could be done to prevent a future heart attack:

> Well, I was not worried about having another heart attack. I was worried about either inducing some sort of irregularity or whatever because I'd had a couple of episodes where I'd had some irregularities that they had to deal with. I was primarily worried that I might strain the heart muscle and hurt the healing process or whatever. Those were my major concerns. . . . Even though we were reading a lot, I still didn't understand all the functions of the heart and all the things you could do that might do something about that.

In order to regain a sense of control the informants used a variety of strategies to minimize uncertainty, including gauging their progress, seeking reassurance, learning about the heart, and practicing cautiousness. All of these strategies were directed toward the minimization of uncertainty. If the informants were able to successfully minimize their uncertainty, then they felt a sense of control; and until a sense of control was regained the informants were unable to start "living again."

Gauging Progress

The informants in this study were able to minimize their sense of uncertainty if they felt they were making progress. Gauging their progress was extremely important to the functions because it provided proof that they were recovering from the heart attack:

> When you look back at it and you say, "Hey, I did this and that and I got away with it, and I slept like a log, and I didn't get angina, I didn't have to take nitro," you feel good don't you? And you can say, "I'm getting better because I can do all these things." And you feel good about it. . . . In a way, you've got to have gauges. You really have got to have them.

Most of the informants desperately wanted to believe that they would fully recover: "I just have got to somehow get the feeling in my head that I'm okay." The informants used a variety of methods to gauge their progress, including goal setting, reviewing their progress, and making comparisons with others. Usually, the method favored by the informant provided the strongest proof of improvement.

All of the informants engaged in goal setting of some kind. They believed that if they could set goals and work toward the accomplishment of these goals they would be able to determine that they were indeed improving. The ways varied in which the informants set these goals. Many would set up daily goals and attempt to meet them. Attempting to meet daily goals not only provided the informants with a means of gauging progress, it also supplied a structure to what was considered a boring existence: "I set little goals for myself each day and try to get them all done. Even though it is nothing, it's something for me."

Initially, most of the informants had difficulty developing realistic goals as they were unsure about what they could realistically accomplish:

> I think initially I was extremely disappointed because, don't forget, I
> thought I was doing fine until I got into the real world of cold air. And
> now I've got to go from A to B. Before, in the hallways at the hospital,
> you've got no place you have to go. When I got home, I said, "I'll walk
> down to Al's house today" or something. And you find out you can only
> make it halfway. You've set a target, and you sure can't meet that target.
> So you've lost your target, and you think, "My God, is this as far as I'm
> going to go."

Once the informants established a baseline for their abilities they
were able to set realistic goals. And once the informants had set
realistic goals the meeting of a goal was viewed as a victory; and
these victories provided the informants with a feeling of "satisfaction
and accomplishment."

The establishment of goals provided some of the informants with
a sense of accomplishment because they helped to structure the
rehabilitation period. By working toward goals they were able to
establish some direction and purpose in their lives: "What's the
purpose of getting up in the morning unless you've got something
to get up for and something to do, to think about, somewhere to go."

Although the informants who were uncertain about the future had
difficulty establishing goals, once these individuals sensed some
improvement in their health, their attitude toward the future became
more positive:

> I could see every single day that I went out walking [that] I was better than
> the day before. And I could tell with the rapid improvement in most of my
> physical signs that if I could do that much in a week I was going to get
> better. Suddenly, I didn't feel very invalid-like anymore. In three or four
> weeks, I could see my physical progress increase so rapidly that I began
> to believe that maybe I was going to be okay. . . . That victory reinforced
> the fact that I was probably going to be able to lead pretty much a normal
> life the rest of my life.

For these individuals their ability to set goals increased as their
self-evaluations improved. Once they believed they had a future they
were willing to take steps to structure and gauge their progress.

The most difficult goals to establish and meet were long-term
goals. The majority of informants felt that they should "take things
one day at a time" and were reluctant to make long-term goals. Those
who engaged in long-term goal setting were often disappointed.

Many of these goals were based on information provided to the informants by health professionals. Some informants would take information about the healing of the heart and interpret it to mean that they would be well in a certain period of time. For example, one informant believed that she should be back to normal in three months because this was the period of time that she believed it would take the heart to heal. When the three month anniversary of her heart attack passed and she was still unable to resume her previous pace of activities, she became extremely disappointed:

> They said your heart is supposed to be healed in eight to twelve weeks, so I believed it. I said, "Well, I'll be home free. Then I can do whatever I want." . . . I've changed my goals so often now there's no use setting them really. There's no use pounding the post too hard. You've got to be able to move it.

The purpose of the informants' goal setting was to gauge their recovery progress. If goals were repeatedly not met the informants became extremely discouraged and stopped setting goals.

Reviewing their progress toward resuming normal activities was a second method used by the informants to gauge their recovery. This method of gauging progress was related to goal setting in that it provided the informants with a sense of accomplishment and improvement; however, it did not necessitate the formal establishment of goals. Through this review the informants were able to gauge how much progress they had made in the previous weeks; in turn, this provided evidence that they were recovering from the heart attack. Time was a great healer for many of the informants. The answer to unmet goals was often "give it time." Time also provided proof of improvement. For example, one informant, who was afraid to leave the hospital, remembered thinking, "Gee, I've been home from the hospital for a week and nothing's happened. I must be okay." Another informant also described the importance of time:

> As time goes on, you just realize you are improving. I was just thinking, well, on the second of April it was exactly three months since I got my heart attack, and I am getting stronger and stronger. I can remember when it was just two weeks after I'd got out of the hospital, and I couldn't hardly do anything. I can feel myself little by little all the time just getting a little stronger.

The progress that was not readily apparent to the informants became clearer through a review of their progress toward resuming normal activities. Through this process, small improvements took on larger dimensions. For example, the informants thought being able to walk two blocks was a large improvement when they considered that just two weeks before it had been difficult to walk to the bathroom and back. Even those informants who were experiencing a great deal of difficulty with the adjustment process could review their progress and find some reason to be positive about the future. Initially the simple act of being discharged from the hospital constituted a form of progress; however, it was important for the process of review to include a gauge of progress over time. If the informants felt stalled in their recovery from the heart attack they would cease the process of reviewing their progress toward a normal life.

The final method of gauging progress was to make comparisons with others in order to remind themselves that their situation could be worse. Using this method the informants attempted to find a candidate, preferably with cardiac disease, who was worse off than themselves. Accordingly, they made comparisons between themselves and this other individual. This in turn provided a gauge of progress as it reminded them of how much they had improved and that their situation could be worse. Every informant made comparisons of this nature, and the only criterion for selection of an individual for comparison was that he or she was deemed worse off than the informant. This method of gauging progress was highly effective:

> You start to wonder if you're the only one that's like this or like that, and you talk to them and sit in the coffee room and talk like "How was your heart attack? And what can you do now? And then somebody says they're taking eight kinds of pills now, and you think, "My God, I'm a lot better off than you are." You make yourself feel good. . . . You realize that there are other things that can be a lot worse.

By far the most popular place for making comparisons was in the cardiac rehabilitation classes. As the informants became veterans of the cardiac rehabilitation programs they compared themselves to the newcomers because it served as a strong reminder of the progress they had made:

There was a new girl in the exercise class. She was in the bathroom hooking up the monitor thing. She didn't know how to do it, so I was showing her how to do it, and she said, "Oh, I don't know. This is my first day at exercise. It might be too hard. It mightn't be any good." And I said, "Believe me, it's good." I saw how scared she was, and I realized how far I'd come.

If the informants were unable to identify someone in the cardiac rehabilitation classes for comparison, they often chose individuals with other diseases. Once they believed "it could be worse" they were able to examine their own situations with a different attitude. Consequently, comparisons provided evidence that things "were not so bad":

There I am feeling useless, and there is my daughter-in-law's mother in just about the same situation with M.S. [multiple sclerosis]. At least I could look forward to getting better, whereas this lady couldn't. This lady could look forward to getting worse. It kind of shook me up. It stopped me from feeling sorry for myself. It kind of says, "Hey, just a minute here. You're not as bad off as you think you are. It could be worse."

I would be a lot more concerned if it had been a spinal injury or a stroke. . . . I'm glad it was a heart attack instead of a stroke. If I had to have one or the other, I'd rather go for the heart attack any day of the week.

The method of making comparisons allowed the informants to consider their conditions in a new light, and their heart condition took on a different meaning once the informants made these comparisons. This gauge provided a meaningful way for the informants to assess their conditions positively, and in turn these positive self-evaluations enabled the informants to minimize their uncertainty.

Seeking Reassurance

Seeking reassurance was the second strategy used by the informants to minimize uncertainty. If the informants were uncertain about their progress, their abilities, or their futures, they attempted to alleviate this uncertainty by seeking reassurance. Reassurance was primarily sought from health care professionals as it was believed that they were the only ones who "knew what they were talking about." A professional opinion was deemed to have greater value than the opinion of a lay person. A second source of support that was extremely important to all of the informants was the reassurance they received from other heart attack victims.

Reassurance was important because it helped alleviate the informants' fears of the unknown. By far the greatest form of reassurance was provided through the cardiac rehabilitation programs. All of the informants believed that these programs "gave you confidence." This was extremely important because the informants were unsure of their abilities when they returned home: "You need the program to train you. If you leave it to your own judgment, you might do something wrong because you're a poor judge." The rehabilitation programs provided the informants with a safe environment for testing their limits:

> They push you to your limit, but they're right there. Like, you have the confidence in them that you're not going to do anything that you shouldn't be doing. They watch you. They know what's happening to you.

In addition, many of the informants believed that the presence of health care professionals protected them from making errors in judgment. As a result, they were able to relax their attempts at reestablishing control when health professionals were present to care for them. Most of the informants felt that without the assistance of the cardiac rehabilitation program staff they would have done something "wrong":

> You could do everything wrong if you start on your own right away, if you're not put into a properly run class. I think that's very important. Because you put on the pasties [cardiac monitor electrodes] and the girl [nurse] watches you on the scope [cardiac monitor], and if something goes wrong, and things do go wrong once in a while, she stops you or the person that it's happening to and says, "You better stop for a moment" or "You better quit for today."

Many of the informants said that when they were at the cardiac rehabilitation center they were able to forgo the responsibility for their health problems. This was the only setting in which they could "let down their guard," not because they no longer required a sense of control but because they felt that in this situation the responsibility for monitoring and maintaining control could be safely handled by others. They felt they could relax their vigilance as someone else was present to take responsibility: "It is their problem if they make me work too hard. If I fall down, they are there to pick me up. So it was out of my hands, and that made me stronger."

The informants also used health care professionals as sources of reassurance regarding their progress. They sought this reassurance in order to allay fears that they were not doing well. The informants were assured they were doing well when health care professionals concurred with their evaluations; however, they were troubled if the assessments they received from health care professionals did not agree with their own evaluation. Figure 2.6 provides a schematic representation of the possible outcomes that could occur when the informants sought professional reassurance. Cell *a* (Figure 2.6) represents those individuals who believe that they are doing well. This belief is present when the informant's perception of his or her progress agrees with the health professionals' evaluation.

Cell *b* (Figure 2.6) represents the informants who felt they were doing well but believed the health care professionals held a different opinion. These individuals described themselves as "devastated":

> Yesterday, you should have talked to me, I was really optimistic. Now today, they took it all away. I thought I was really doing great. . . . I don't know, I always get this pounding feeling, but it doesn't bother me, and I just thought it is something that will go away. I thought I had it pretty well licked. . . . I thought I had it by the tail. Now, I don't know what to think or do.

Once the informants believed they were getting well any negative insinuations devastated them. This incongruency shattered their belief in their ability to judge their progress. One informant described the disagreement between her evaluation of her progress and a health care professional's evaluation as "a huge let down." Once the informants lost faith in their powers of judgment they felt incapable of making decisions; in turn, this loss of faith heightened their sense of a loss of control. These individuals found that they had to rethink the meaning of their heart attack, and in order to understand their present situation they were forced to return to the process of making sense of the event. Many of the informants who

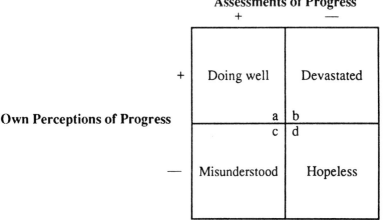

Figure 2.6. Perceptions of Progress

experienced this devastation considered the future tentative, and they reconsidered their initial optimistic or positive attitudes.

Those individuals whose self-evaluations were negative and who believed that the health care professionals' assessments were positive are depicted in Cell *c* (Figure 2.6). They believed that their problems were not properly understood by the health care team and they were generally distrustful of the evaluations of the physicians and nurses. Generally, these informants lacked confidence and they were unwilling to believe that they were doing well. They described themselves as "misunderstood." Symptoms such as weakness and fatigue were of great concern to them; however, when they described these symptoms to their physicians and nurses they felt they were merely placated. They were unable to accept that their symptoms were typical. As a result they lost faith in the established health care system. These individuals were torn between a fear that they were experiencing serious symptoms and a need to be reassured. This conflict was only resolved when the informants were able to establish some agreement between their self-evaluations and the evaluations made by health care providers.

Those individuals whose self-evaluations were negative and who believed that health care professionals supported this assessment are depicted in Cell *d* (Figure 2.6). These individuals described themselves as "hopeless." They believed that little could be done to improve their condition. One informant, who initially thought she was doing well, came to believe that the health care professionals thought she was doing poorly. As a result of this conflict she modified her self-evaluation to match what she perceived to be the health care professionals' assessment. She became hopeless about her future, believing that little could be done to improve her health.

Seeking reassurance did not always help the informants minimize their uncertainty. In some cases, if they did not get the positive assessment they were looking for seeking reassurance only increased the informants' sense of uncertainty. Although most of the informants did not want to discuss the disagreement between their evaluations of their progress and the health care professionals' evaluations, it is important to note the factors that led the informants to believe that health care professionals held "negative evaluations" of their progress. Generally, any comment that was not blatantly positive was considered negative. In one situation a physician ordered additional tests for an informant, and the informant interpreted this to mean that she was not progressing, that something was wrong. Many of the informants were emotionally fragile during their first six weeks at home, and they desperately sought signs of hope from members of the health care team. When these signs were not readily apparent they became discouraged.

Although the opinions of health care professionals were highly valued by the informants, reassurance was also received from other heart attack victims. For the informants in this study the support and advice of others who had also experienced a heart attack was extremely reassuring. "Having somebody to talk to who has been through it" was considered an invaluable source of support. The cardiac rehabilitation classes were ideal places for finding support of this nature:

> Those classes are good. You see everybody in the same boat, and you talk about it, and you begin to learn that it's not so bad. You think that you're the only one it ever happened to. My God. And you find out you're not the only one in the world who has had their life upset.

The reassurance gained by watching others cope successfully with their heart attacks was invaluable to the informants, and this form of reassurance was less threatening as the informants felt free to reject the opinion of other lay persons and seek advice elsewhere.

Learning About the Heart

Learning about the heart was a third strategy used by the informants to minimize their uncertainty. Most of the informants said they knew little about the heart prior to their heart attacks, and many of them believed that an understanding of the heart enabled them to understand "what was happening" to them. For the informants in this study, learning about the heart was considered extremely important as it made the event and the rehabilitation more manageable:

> Understanding what's happened is 90% of the battle. If you don't understand, you're going to be scared. . . . You're only scared of what you don't know. Even when I was a little wee kid and left alone in the house, if I heard sounds around, instead of hiding in the dark, I'd open the bedroom window so that if there was something out there I could see it. Once I saw it, or saw there was nothing, the fear would go away. But as long as you stayed and hid in the dark from it, then you're scared 'cause anything could be there, right? . . . So knowing what's happened is very important.

Information about the heart provided some of the informants with a sense of control. To understand what was happening gave them the control they needed to plan for the future and predict outcomes: "I'm a person who wants to know exactly what is going on. I don't care whether it's good news or bad news. I just need to know intellectually what the hell is happening." An understanding of what a heart attack is enabled some of the informants to make sense of what remained unclear about their own condition. When asked what he thought about learning about the heart, one informant said, "I think I've finally grasped enough that I will take a warning now. I won't let it get off my back." Another informant said,

> I want to know the mechanisms that are going on, how the whole thing functions, the works. And if I don't understand, then there are pieces missing in my mind, then I don't have any strategy for coping with it.

The importance of learning about the heart varied among the informants. Although a need to understand what was happening was expressed by all of the informants, some believed that knowledge of the heart would not help them understand their heart condition:

> I just wonder why it does that. I would like to know. She explained all about how, you know, there's two parts to the beat and . . . the damage is all at the bottom so it should set up signals, a couple here and there where it's not supposed to be, but it doesn't really make sense to me. . . . And I keep thinking, "What's wrong?" They don't really tell you what's wrong, just how it does it. And there's a difference.

Many of the informants who felt that knowledge of the heart was not particularly helpful had difficulty relating to the abstract nature of the heart and information about cardiac physiology and anatomy did not aid them in understanding what was happening to their particular heart.

Many of the informants said they wanted to know specifically what had happened to their heart. Generalities about what caused heart attacks were not sufficient for these individuals. They wanted to know exactly "what the damage was"; however, they discovered that health care professionals were unwilling to provide this information:

> I would like to know exactly what happened to my heart. It's important to know about it because then it's not so scary. I specifically, point blank asked them about it, and they wouldn't tell me. They said it didn't matter. I don't know if it would do me any good, but I'd still like to know.

When asked why knowledge about her heart was so important, one informant said, "I don't know. Just maybe it would change the way I feel about myself or something. Maybe it would help me understand what level I will be at."

Learning about the heart enabled the informants to understand what had happened to their hearts. Although this strategy enabled some informants to develop an understanding upon which decisions could be based, others felt threatened by information about the heart. This strategy was deemed useful only when the information received was believed to be helpful. Although information was important to all of the informants, the amount and type of information believed to be helpful differed between informants.

Knowledge of the roles that diet, exercise, and rest play in the rehabilitation process was helpful to all of the informants. Many of them expressed a need to have clear guidelines for what and what not to do, and they wanted all the answers in "black and white." Information of this nature provided the informants with guidance about how to live their lives, and it also served to minimize their uncertainty.

Two of the informants said that at times knowledge about the heart made them anxious. Rather than alleviating their uncertainties they found that knowledge about the heart and the symptoms of heart disease sensitized them to the possibilities of what could go wrong.

> The things that I would not even probably consider before or not even consciously be aware of, these little things inside, all of the sudden you are aware because it's brought to your attention. . . . I think maybe the less you know, it's better for you.

These individuals tended to become preoccupied with the possibilities of reoccurring symptoms. For example, following a teaching session that focused on angina one informant said she spent the next week worrying about whether she was experiencing angina. She said that she became uncomfortably self-conscious as she feared that "every little twinge" was an angina attack.

Practicing Cautiousness

Practicing cautiousness was the final strategy used by the informants to minimize their uncertainty. This strategy was used to ensure that they did not harm themselves by overactivity, and it was practiced when an informant was feeling vulnerable and "out of control." All of the informants expressed concerns regarding the possibility of "overdoing it." They were afraid that any form of overexertion could potentially cause serious health problems:

> Well, I'm scared of the angina, you know, because I did have it, and I keep on thinking, "Will I have another heart attack?" So I keep on thinking, "Well, if I do things slowly and get back into the swing of it slowly, I won't have one."

Although all of the informants believed that the way to prevent another heart attack was to avoid overdoing it, the informants practiced cautiousness in a variety of ways. The degree to which an individual used the strategy of practicing cautiousness depends on the extent to which he or she felt in control. For example, informants believed that they did not have to be as cautious in cardiac rehabilitation classes because health care professionals maintained vigilance for them; whereas they believed that they had to be extremely cautious when engaging in activities that had not been performed since the time of the heart attack.

Many of the informants expressed concern about the resumption of activities following their heart attacks. Although they did not want to overexert themselves, they wanted to push themselves toward improvement:

> So you gotta go for as much as you can, but you can't overdo it. . . . Like you don't want to think, "Oh, I can't do that." But then, you don't want to hurt yourself either, so you don't want to do anything to impede your getting well.

Although many of the informants felt that overexertion was to be avoided, they also believed that they should not be "lazy." Consequently, they found it difficult to make decisions regarding an appropriate level of activity. They did not trust their abilities as judges and they were concerned that they might make the wrong decisions. Rather than risk the possibility of hurting themselves, they chose to err on the side of cautiousness.

The practice of cautiousness as a strategy was a conscious effort. Some informants believed that if they did not practice some form of cautiousness, they would automatically overdo things out of habit:

> I was a little worried . . . that I would overdo it. In the hospital, quite unconsciously, I was moving a chair, and I picked it up until I realized, "Oh, I shouldn't be doing this." And you know, I put it down fast. I wasn't feeling too bad when I came home. I was a little scared that I might forget for a little while and then just plow into whatever I was doing.

Many of the informants described situations in which they reminded themselves to take it easy.

All of the informants said that rather than engage in a task that could lead to a questionable outcome they would choose not to do it. The informants avoided "taking any chances." In turn, this strategy ensured that the informants maintained control. For some of the informants these decisions were not difficult to make. For others every new task was approached with a sense of cautiousness. Some of the informants refused to engage in any activity until they had checked with their physicians or nurses. The fear of overexertion had the potential to paralyze some of the informants. These individuals found themselves caught between a desire to "carry on as usual" and a fear that if they did carry on as usual they might hurt themselves and possibly die:

> I'm still going through it, and I think, "Oh, I'm sure I can do this myself," and "Why can't I do it?" I'm scared of overdoing it. I'm worried whether I should have a fear like that. I'm scared to do too much. And what is frustrating is I think, "Well, should I do it, or shouldn't I do it? Why do I have a fear of doing anything until I ask somebody if I can do it?"

For some informants in this study it was difficult to live with the decision to be cautious. They remained fearful that they were not actively attempting to improve, and they felt they were malingering. They believed that they should be doing more, and yet they were afraid of the consequences of increasing their activity levels:

> I was scared that I was a baby. Even when I got home, I thought, "Gee, am I babying myself? Can't I do this?" I was scared that I was babying myself, and I kept on thinking, "Am I too afraid of what I've had?" I think I am, you know?

For some individuals the fear of overexertion and losing control ruled their lives for many months. One informant refused to leave her home unaccompanied for fear that something would happen to her. When questioned about this she said, "I thought, well, if I go out and something happens, I'd be so ashamed." For this informant the strategy of practicing cautiousness was used to protect her self-esteem as well as her physical well-being.

The only strategy that aided the informants in ridding themselves of their uncertainties was to practice some form of cautiousness.

Some of the informants were able to harness the uncertainties they faced early in the adjustment process. Others who were unable to allay their fears continued practicing cautiousness for many months following their heart attacks. This strategy was used until the individual was able to reestablish a sense of predictability and independence: "I can't push myself. It's always at the back of my mind that I shouldn't push, and I'm scared. I'm scared, you know, and it's been over three months."

Establishing Guidelines for Living

As the heart attack victim struggles to preserve a sense of self and minimize uncertainty, he or she must face the challenge of establishing guidelines for living. Before these individuals are able to regain a sense of control they must find ways to restructure their lives. The life of the heart attack victim is unalterably changed. Fear, uncertainty, and physical symptoms undermine one's sense of control. A heart attack disrupts plans and disorganizes the day-to-day structure of an individual's life. The heart attack victim is faced with the task of reordering his or her life. This objective is accomplished through the establishment of guidelines; and through the establishment of guidelines for living, the heart attack victim reestablishes a sense of control.

Every individual requires some guidelines for living. Although these guidelines are not necessarily formal, they provide a sense of structure and control. In the absence of guidelines an individual is faced with absolute uncertainty. Guidelines for living include an understanding of corporal limitations and an understanding of how one's life will be lived. The day-to-day functions of living are all performed within guidelines. Individuals usually attempt to avoid situations that will cause them harm. Guidelines for living provide a structure for making these judgments. The establishment of guidelines orders an individual's life and therefore enhances his or her sense of predictability, independence, and self-determination.

The informants in this study described three strategies that they used to establish guidelines for living: testing their limitations, learning to read their bodies, and modifying their life-styles. The heart attack totally disrupted the plans and the rhythms of the informants' lives, and all of these strategies were directed toward the reestablishment of control.

Testing Limitations

As the informants gained confidence in their abilities, they began to test their limitations. Each new activity was approached with trepidation and the once normal routines of their lives were viewed as challenges. Initially most of the informants faced new challenges with a sense of cautiousness; however, as they progressed in the adjustment process they began to test their abilities. While the informants practiced cautiousness in order to cognitively maintain a sense of control, they tested limitations in order to reestablish a sense of physical control and mastery. Many of the informants said they had to engage in each activity at least once before they felt comfortable with a particular activity:

> There was a bit of apprehension about driving. . . . So you always want to see whether you can do it. That, I think, is the whole thing: "Can I do it?" If I do it once and it doesn't cause me any problem, I can go back and do it again.

Driving a car, having sex, bowling, vacuuming, and going out are examples of challenges that had to be tested and overcome. As abilities were tested, the informants felt their limits were being "stretched":

> Like, I wouldn't do anything stupid. I wouldn't try anything that I knew I couldn't do or keep doing something that was beyond my limits. But I think you can keep getting your limits, you can stretch them, and you can keep stretching them until your limits go pretty far.

Many of the informants consciously attempted to challenge themselves as they believed this was the only way to overcome their limits. Testing their limitations in this way contributed to their sense of progress. It also reinforced their confidence in their abilities. Without this testing many of the informants believed they would "stagnate":

> I've got to always say to myself, "Hey, I betcha I can do that and get away with it." You know, you have to, and I'm doing it all the time. I think a lot of people do this. How in the heck do you know what you can do if you don't try?

The testing the informants engaged in was based on their perceptions of what they should be able to accomplish; in turn, this testing enabled them to gain a sense of confidence.

Some of the informants said that at times they pushed "too hard" in their attempts to extend their limitations. Testing of this nature was conducted in order to prove their abilities to themselves and others: "You go out, and you push yourself sometimes when you shouldn't. You do this because it proves you can still do it and that you're not an invalid anymore." The informants were extremely disappointed when they tested their limits and were unable to meet their goals. Often they would be reluctant to resume testing until they resolved their feeling of being disabled. When the results of the testing were uncertain the informants avoided testing their limits as it held the potential for failure.

Testing limits continued until the informants were able to regain a sense of mastery and no longer required a conscious test of their abilities. Positive results from the testing of their limitations resulted in an affirmation of their abilities. Limitations which were initially assumed by the informants were disproved by testing limits. By testing their limits those informants who initially believed that they would be faced with a permanent disability were often able to prove to themselves that many of their assumed limitations did not exist. In turn this prompted them to reconsider the possibilities for their future. Informants who began to disprove their restrictions returned to the stage of making sense of the event and began to evaluate their future in a positive manner:

> I thought it would be too hard, but now I don't think so. Before, like after I had the heart attack, I thought I might feel good again, but I didn't ever think really good. Like now, I think I feel really good. And I think I'll feel even better. Like before, I felt probably there would be some restriction in my life forever, but I don't think so anymore.

Testing limits enabled the informants to determine what they could and could not do. Many of the informants faced some form of restriction following their heart attacks. For example, they could not work as hard or as long as they once did or they found activities such as dancing or golfing difficult. They believed that they needed to determine their abilities in order to know when to say "no" and when to quit:

You have to know your limits. If you go ahead and do things, certainly know your limits. If you are getting too exhausted, too tired, well just sit down. If you don't know your limits, you may never do anything, or you may overdo it.

The testing of limitations enabled the informants to regain a sense of predictability and independence, and they learned how to pace themselves. These lessons were only learned through the trial and error testing of their limitations.

Learning to Read One's Body

Learning to read one's body is a strategy closely related to the strategy of testing limitations. Many of the informants believed that they were unable to trust their abilities following their heart attacks. They had difficulty determining how much activity was appropriate. In order to overcome this barrier, they were faced with the task of learning to trust their body's abilities. This was accomplished by becoming sensitized to the body's needs and demands. Many of the informants said they were out of touch with what was happening to their bodies, and the fact that they had experienced a sudden and traumatic event was used by the informants as proof that they were out of touch with their bodies.

Many of the informants said that prior to their heart attack they did not respect their body's signals to slow down. For example, despite symptoms of fatigue they would drive themselves to complete tasks. The heart attack was an event that caused them to consider the fragility of the body. Many of them believed that they needed to be in "better touch" with their bodies, but this was a difficult task as they had not previously considered their physical needs.

For the informants, the major sign of overexertion was angina. At times it was difficult for the informants to learn about the symptoms that constitute angina. Many lived with a fear that they would experience angina and not recognize it. The subtlety of angina was extremely confusing and many of the informants were afraid they would not immediately recognize symptoms such as jaw pain, neck pain, and heartburn. Consequently, it often took several bouts of angina before the informants felt comfortable recognizing and treating it:

You didn't know how you would know that the angina pain really comes and how it affects you. Like, even when I felt a certain pain, I sort of discounted it, that maybe it wasn't an angina pain. But it was, you see? It's difficult to adjust. It is an adjustment that you have to go through to realize what an angina pain is really like.

Those informants who did not experience angina following their heart attacks initially lived in fear that they would not be able to recognize it should it occur: "You have maybe pains or whatever in your body and whatever sensations, and you don't know what they are. Are they something to be concerned about or are they not?" Some of the informants experienced a hypersensitivity to their bodies and they scrutinized every sensation. As time passed these individuals began to believe that they would not experience angina; consequently, they developed confidence in their ability to read their bodies and they were able to focus their attention on other aspects of their lives.

The informants also had to learn to be aware of symptoms such as fatigue and shortness of breath. An understanding of their body's needs and abilities provided the informants with a means by which they could measure their limitations and abilities:

Occasionally, I was wondering whether I should or shouldn't do my gardening work. But it seemed that I could trust my body to tell me that's enough for now, and then I would quit.

Some of the informants in this study became extremely active in monitoring their abilities. They monitored their pulse rates and adjusted their medications to meet their needs. They developed a sensitivity to changes in their bodies, and in turn they developed confidence in their abilities to read and control their symptoms. These particular informants indicated that accurately reading the body gave them a sense of control:

It took me . . . at least three months to run enough experiments on myself to figure out how to regulate my medicine, how to regulate my eating, how to regulate my other daily habits to where I have 99% of the time no problems of any kind. I never have angina or anything. If I want to have angina, I can have it, but I've learned how to avoid it.

The informants' sensitivity to their body's abilities enabled them to develop a sense of trust, and this sensitivity provided them with a means by which they could make judgments regarding the continuation of an activity:

> You've got to know your warnings. There are things that if you do them and don't listen to the warnings you will overstep your bounds. The doctor puts certain limitations on you, but they're too general. You've got to figure out for yourself what your body can do.

The informants' ability to read and trust their bodies was developed over time. This strategy was used in combination with the strategy of testing their limitations. Before limits were tested the informants required some ability in reading the body. Once they had this ability the limitation testing provided feedback about their ability to read their bodies.

Modifying Life-Style

Modifying their life-style was the final strategy that the informants in this study used to establish guidelines for living. The modification of life-styles is not simply a strategy that involves making and implementing decisions regarding life-style changes; rather, this strategy involves the serious consideration of life-style changes, attempts to implement and evaluate life-style changes, and, if the outcomes are positive, the incorporation of these changes into one's life. The strategy of making life-style modifications is complex. Not only do decisions about life-style have an impact on the individual, they also have an impact on the individual's entire family.

Decisions regarding life-style modifications are structured by the way in which the individual made sense of his or her heart attack:

> It was stress that caused my heart attack. I understand now what causes stress, and I'm very conscious of the fact that stress can bring another problem back. So I'm learning to avoid the situation that caused the stress.

Those individuals who did not experience the improvements that they expected as a result of their life-style modifications returned to the task of making sense of the heart attack. These informants sought other causal explanations and they attempted other life-style modifications.

One informant believed that his heart attack was due to the stress he had experienced at work. Although he was 55 years old and had been informed that he would be able to return to work, he chose to retire. He believed that returning to work would be returning to the problem that caused his heart attack. This informant reassessed his life goals as a result of his heart attack. Having been exposed to a life threatening event, he decided that he should attempt to live life to its fullest. He wanted to enjoy his life and spend time with his family. Although others might view his decision to retire as indicative of a rehabilitation failure, he said his choice was motivated by something other than fear or a belief that he was crippled. He was motivated by the belief that only through retirement could his life be lived to its fullest.

All of the informants indicated that life-style changes should be gradual as a "total life adjustment" cannot be implemented quickly. The changes considered particularly difficult were those that involved changes in attitude. One informant said it was impossible to change as he could not "reprogram his mind." The best he believed he could do was to modify his current life-style. The majority of the informants indicated that although it was important to gradually make modifications to their life-styles it was also important to believe in the implemented changes. Those informants who attempted to "force" themselves to change inevitably failed to sustain the changes. To attempt changes that they believed would not make a difference to their health "set [them] up for failure."

In this study there were interesting contrasts between the ways in which the male and female informants made life-style modifications. The majority of the men considered the modification of their life-styles to be a joint venture between themselves and their spouses. The male informants spoke of the changes in terms of "we." In particular, the older men expected their wives to attend cardiac rehabilitation classes and learn to cook "for them":

[My wife has] entered the classes there, and she is monitoring my diet, and I think I've started to lose weight. Diet is her responsibility because I don't even know how to boil an egg. So as I say, she's looking after that.

The women in this study tended to make life-style changes independently. They did not involve their spouses to the same extent as the men, and these differences were noticed by the female
informants:

> You know, the men I speak with at the classes . . . just assume that their
> wives will come along to the classes so they can learn to cook for them.
> But the women who've had heart attacks don't assume that their husbands
> will come along, you know. . . . I think once I saw a husband down there
> at one of the lectures.

The women also took sole responsibility for their dietary changes
and they were generally reluctant to make changes they thought
might negatively affect their families. Many prided themselves in
their ability to cook and they were unwilling to sacrifice recipes that
contained ingredients high in cholesterol or calories, particularly if
their family members enjoyed eating them. Most of them attempted
to modify their favorite recipes; however, this was not always successful. Family members often noticed the lack of salt in the cooking
and the absence of fried foods and sweets; consequently, this created
a conflict. On one hand, the women wanted to modify their life-
styles; and on the other hand, they did not want their family members
to "suffer" because of them. Those who were able to resolve this
conflict did so because they believed they were providing their
families with "good" nutrition.

Generally, the life-style modifications the female informants incorporated into their lives were done surreptitiously so as not to disrupt
their families' routines. The women were concerned about the ex-
pense of making dietary changes and the time involved in cardiac
rehabilitation programs; however, the men in this study did not voice
concerns of this nature.

Over the course of time the informants began to view the life-style
modifications they had made as permanent. Life-style modifications
had to be considered a part of the informants' lives before they were
able to state that they had truly made modifications. Many believed
that in order to incorporate these changes they had to be "tested"
first. Testing involved being confronted with temptations and making selections that were consistent with their new life-styles. Settings

in which this testing took place included the work site, restaurants, and social gatherings. If the informants could sustain their new life-styles in the face of these challenges, they believed they were "home free." One informant did not feel he would be tested until he returned to work. He had resolved not to take on every problem at work that came to his attention, and he believed that the only way in which he would be able to test his resolve would be to actually experience an extremely stressful situation. Over the course of repeated testing, the modifications that the informants made became "a part of living."

Stage Four: Living Again

As the informants struggled through the adjustment process they were often confronted with the fact that they were not living life to its fullest. During the initial stages all of their efforts were directed toward the reestablishment of control. Once a sense of control was reestablished, they were able to begin to live again: "It takes a while to build up your confidence, and then you basically have to start living all over again." Gradually the informants entered this final stage of the adjustment process, the living again phase. As the informants regained a sense of control they began to refocus their attention on other aspects of life. The heart attack was no longer their primary concern. Although the informants never forgot that they had experienced a heart attack, as the final stage of the adjustment process was reached they were able to place the event behind them and focus on other aspects of their lives.

One informant described himself as a "car on the highway who's having the carbon blown out." Although this informant initially believed he would never improve, he was able to regain a sense of control in his life and come to terms with his limitations. Most of the informants were unable to point out when they began to "get on with life." One informant suggested that she was living again when she said, "I feel like a whole person again. I know what I can do. I can do what everybody else does. I can do what I did before." There were three responses that characterized this stage: an acceptance of one's limitations, a refocusing on other concerns and issues, and an attainment of a sense of mastery. These three responses were the hallmarks of the final stage as they provided a strong indication that the individual was no longer struggling with the adjustment process:

> You feel good in so many ways, you really do. Now I get the bicycle out, and I just love it. I just get on that bicycle and go like hell. I go further and further all the time. And I know the old heart won't quit on me. I don't even think about it.

Accepting Limitations

Many of the informants were faced with some form of limitation following their heart attacks. Following a testing period the informants were faced with the task of accepting their limitations, and this acceptance was often gradual. Some of the informants said they appreciated the limitations that had been imposed upon them because they had discovered new aspects of life as a result of being "forced" to slow down: "I don't push like I used to. If I feel I want to sit down and have a cup of tea, that's what I do. And you know, I enjoy it."

Often the informants would change their expectations in order to incorporate their new limitations into their lives. By decreasing or changing their expectations the informants eliminated their sense of limitation. The informants accomplished this by reexamining their goals and expectations and by reconsidering their priorities:

> It used to annoy me for things to be messy, but I've learned to take things in my stride. I've had to let go of certain things. I've learned how to not let it bother me if the kitchen floor doesn't get washed. I've had to. Other things are more important.

Eventually the limitations that the informants experienced were incorporated into their lives to such an extent that they were no longer considered limitations. Ultimately they were considered a part of living. The limitations that were once perceived to be insurmountable were now "taken in stride":

> I've finally realized that it is okay to curb some of my activities. I'm 64 years old, and I've got to start slowing down. I'm still alert and very progressive, but I've got a physical requirement that is forcing me to slow down a bit, and that's alright.

Many of the informants believed that once they had learned to pace themselves limitations were no longer insurmountable: "You're always at a decided disadvantage compared to other people. However, it is a problem which I have learned to live with." This change in attitude provided the informants with a new sense of control. They began to believe that the task of living could be accomplished; perhaps more slowly, perhaps not in the same way as before, but nonetheless they could go on living. Consequently, the informants were able to minimize the uncertainties of the future.

Refocusing

As the informants accepted their limitations they began to refocus their attention on other aspects of life. The heart attack was no longer the informants' primary concern. This refocusing was due to the control that was reestablished: "The uncertainties are gradually fading away. I mean, there will always be worries, but just not so pronounced." Much of the refocusing was enhanced by the passage of time. As the months passed the perceived severity of the heart attack diminished:

> You're feeling great. You can do these things. You're confident of yourself, and so it doesn't seem there are things to be uncertain about. It takes time. It doesn't matter what anybody preaches at you.

> I think the farther down the road you get with your own rehabilitation the easier it gets to take. Things concern you less. You are able to put things in perspective. Basically, I've learned to put what's happened behind me.

The refocusing was enhanced by the informants' physical improvements. Physical limitations such as weakness and fatigue diminished over time, and a sense of physical improvement enhanced the informants' sense of control and allowed them the freedom to address other concerns in their lives: "You know if you feel good there is nothing nagging at your brain. Then your whole outlook is better. You can feel a little more daring as time goes on."

The third factor that enabled the informants to refocus their attention on other aspects of their lives was their will to live. Many of the informants described dreams and goals that they had yet to fulfill.

They were determined to avoid allowing their lives to be consumed by their heart attacks. They described a desire to live life to its fullest. In some cases this desire was enhanced by the experience of a close brush with death. Those informants who had resolved to "live life differently" in the initial stages of the adjustment process were often driven by this resolution. In one situation this desire to live differently prompted the informant to focus his energy on things and individuals other than himself:

> Oh, my outlook on life has certainly changed. I try and appreciate other people now. I try and look at them and appreciate their concerns, put them first before me. . . . Sometimes I was pretty headstrong in my own selfish ways, but now I just look at people a little differently, with maybe a little bit more love than I did in the past.

Despite this informant's attempt to focus on others his desire was initially thwarted because he had not fully adjusted to his loss of control. Later in the adjustment process he found that he was unable to sustain his attempts to care for others. He discovered that he had to spend time and effort caring for himself before he could effectively redirect his concern toward others.

Attaining Mastery

Attaining a sense of mastery was the final response indicating the successful attainment of the final stage of the adjustment process. Mastery involves an effortless ability to complete tasks without consideration; it is not a self-conscious response. The informants acquired a sense of mastery over time and described mastery in terms of the feelings it provoked, such as "satisfaction," "feelings of accomplishment," "strength," and "pride."

With a sense of mastery the informants were able to carry out the tasks of everyday life without effort. Rather than consider every activity, the selection of tasks was made without conscious effort and a sense of predictability was restored:

> I feel like I've got over the hurdle. I'm able to do things. It gives me a good feeling. The cautiousness is going away. I run up and down the stairs now without even thinking about it. I never used to do that.

Often a sense of mastery caught the informants unaware. Upon reviewing their progress they were able to point out that they were indeed developing confidence and an ever increasing sense of control. With this increasing sense of mastery the informants found they needed fewer supports and no longer required constant reassurance. They had the ability to make decisions about activities and judge their progress. When they recognized their ability, they became confident:

> At the beginning, you don't know what to do. You don't know how far you should go on your own. And then, after a while, you need less help, and basically, you don't want any more help. You feel more freedom without knowing it. You know you are okay. You get a little more space to expand. Your limits broaden out, and you feel comfortable with yourself.

Some of the informants were able to describe moments when they knew they had regained a sense of control in their lives. Certain events were of great significance as they provided strong indicators of their abilities. These accomplishments included activities such as the first time one informant entertained, the efforts one informant made to move boxes, and the completion of a hike up a mountain for another informant:

> I'll tell you one of my happiest times was the summer after I had my heart attack. . . . We went to Banff, to Johnson Canyon . . . and we walked up the mountain there for hours. But I walked careful. I walked easy because I hadn't had my heart attack all that long ago. And I get to about four miles up there, hey, I felt great, and I thought, "God, I'm not a cripple." The last thing you want to be is a cripple. Nobody wants to be. A blind person doesn't want to be blind, and a deaf person doesn't want to be deaf, and a person with a heart attack doesn't want to be a couch potato.

Abandoning the Struggle

There are those individuals who are unable to adjust successfully following a heart attack. These individuals are perpetually caught in the cycle of coming to terms and learning to live and, at times, they find it necessary to abandon the struggle to reestablish control. The individuals who are most likely to abandon the struggle are those who believe that they have experienced "too many" setbacks and believe that the fight to regain control is "hopeless." Heart attack victims are extremely vulnerable to the influence of others and victims' assessments of their improvements are not always accurate. At times individuals can exit from the adjustment process because of a perceived inability to reestablish control. Although somewhat contradictory, the decision to abandon the fight is thought to be the only means by which some semblance of control can be regained. Those individuals who abandon the struggle believe that there is nothing more they can do. Responsibility for the heart attack is surrendered and the heart problems, which they continue to experience, are deemed to be the responsibility of health care providers.

In this study there was one informant who abandoned the struggle to regain control. She experienced numerous setbacks in the adjustment process and she was constantly setting goals and failing to meet them. Eventually, she was no longer able to face perpetual disappointment. She stopped setting goals, refused to monitor her progress, and abandoned attempts to read her body. Her sense of loss repeatedly outweighed any sense of gains:

> It's the doctor's problem. There's nothing I can do about it. Somebody else has got to fix it. I can't. I did all I can. I changed my diet. I quit smoking. I do my exercise. . . . There's no more I can do.

Although there was only one informant in this study who abandoned the struggle to regain control, the other informants expressed a belief that they too would give up if they saw no sign of progress. In fact two other informants exhibited signs of abandoning the fight; however, their situations improved and they were able to reenter the adjustment process. Although the informant who abandoned the fight was by no means the most ill of the informants, she believed that she would not improve. She found that health care professionals working with her provided little sense of hope. When she thought she was doing well she did not believe health care professionals shared her view. She was unable to establish a sense of control over the adjustment process. All attempts to regain control failed; consequently, in order to maintain some semblance of control she stopped trying to regain control. Interviews with this informant spanned a period of six months, and at the time of the last interview she said she had given up. Although her decision is unfortunate, it is possible

that factors may present themselves which would allow this informant the opportunity to reenter the adjustment process.

The Process of Adjustment

The adjustment that individuals experience following a heart attack is a process that incorporates four stages and the ways vary in
which individuals respond to these various stages. Despite this
variation all of the strategies and responses that characterize each
stage of the adjustment process are directed toward regaining a sense
of control.

The largest variation in the adjustment process was found in the
second and third stages, coming to terms with the event and learning
to live. These two stages were found to be highly interrelated.
Although some informants were able to progress smoothly through
the adjustment process from stage to stage, others remained for an
extended period of time in a cycle of making sense of the event and
learning to live. The adjustment process is diagrammatically represented in Figure 2.7. Those individuals who are able to establish and
maintain a positive attitude moved quickly through the adjustment
process. Those individuals who had difficulty establishing or who
were unable to maintain a positive attitude returned several times to
the stage of making sense of the event.

The reflexive nature of the second and third stages of the adjustment process was difficult to uncover. The variation initially described by the informants produced a confusing picture. Not only
was there variation among the informants, but the informants themselves changed their minds and their attitudes over the course of
time. It was the identification of the core category, *regaining control,*
that enabled this investigator to determine the nature of this considerable variation. It was found that all of the responses and strategies
that the informants discussed were directed toward achieving control. The informants made sense of their situations in order to regain
control and it was this understanding that guided their subsequent
responses and selection of strategies:

> You change your mind so many times during the healing process. Like
> you think about the way your life is going, and what you can do. I know
> at one point I thought I would never be able to work again. I was sure I

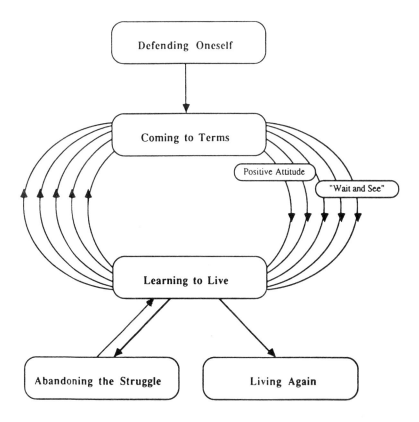

Figure 2.7. The Process of Adjustment Following Heart Attack

couldn't. One day you think you can't do anything. So you don't. The next you think you have the world by the tail. It seems like such a changing process.

All of the informants in this study addressed the different styles of coping they used and witnessed. Many of the informants emphasized the importance of developing a "comfortable style." Certainly, individuals use different styles of adjustment; however, all of the informants directed their efforts of adjustment toward the process of regaining control.

Notes

1. The sample consisted of 14 informants aged 43 to 72 years of age (7 of whom were female) and was composed of two groups: primary informants who had experienced a heart attack within the previous three months, and secondary informants who had experienced a heart attack within the previous four years. The primary informants consisted of individuals enrolled in a cardiac rehabilitation program, and the secondary informants were selected from members of a cardiac self-help group. Each informant was interviewed one to four times.

2. Some of the diagrams and some of the quotations found in this chapter were reprinted with the publisher's permission from: Johnson, J. L., & Morse, J. M. (1990). Regaining control: The process of adjustment after myocardial infarction. *Heart & Lung, 19*, 126-135.

References

Bar-On, D. (1986). Professional models vs. patient models in rehabilitation after heart attack. *Human Relations, 39*, 917-932.

3

The Experiences of Women Having
a Hysterectomy

MARIE ANDRÉE CHASSÉ

One of the strengths of using qualitative methods is that these methods allow the researcher to consider the context of the phenomenon as well as the phenomenon itself. Respecting the context of a phenomenon involves allowing the informants to tell the stories and share the experiences that they believe are relevant. Although Chassé was initially interested in the process of recovery following a hysterectomy, she soon discovered that her informants could not simply discuss their recoveries; rather, they had to discuss all of the events surrounding the hysterectomy beginning with the exacerbation of symptoms and their first hunches that something was wrong. The informants could not separate their recoveries from the initial stages of the hysterectomy decision-making process because part of the recovery process involved resolving the issue of whether they had made the right decision when they consented for surgery. Chassé was sensitive to this fact and incorporated the rich data regarding pre-surgery decision making into her analysis.

Currently, hysterectomy is one of the most frequently performed surgical procedures in North America. Despite advances in surgical procedures and the increasing control of postoperative complica-

AUTHOR'S NOTE: Derived from: Chassé, M. A. (1988). *The experience of women who undergo hysterectomy.* Unpublished master's thesis, University of Alberta, Edmonton, Alberta, Canada.

This research was supported in part by the Alberta Association of Registered Nurses and the Alberta Foundation for Nursing Research.

tions, it is widely recognized that the experiences of women who undergo a hysterectomy are not well understood. Because of its fundamental role in reproduction many social and personal values surround the uterus, and the removal of the uterus may have implications for a woman's emotional and physical well-being. If women are to be adequately supported posthysterectomy their experiences must be understood; therefore, a study was conducted to examine the experiences of women who undergo a hysterectomy.

The experience of women who undergo a hysterectomy was found to be composed of three interdependent stages: the disruption of the body, the struggle to preserve wholeness, and the recovery (Figure 3.1). In the first stage the woman attempts to understand and cope with her health problem; and as she fails in her efforts to manage the symptoms she is faced with the possibility of having a hysterectomy. Eventually, the decision is made to undergo the surgery. During the second stage the woman engages in a struggle to minimize her sense of fragmentation and loss of control. In the third stage the woman begins to adjust to the bodily changes resulting from the hysterectomy and attempts to come to terms with her surgery. Throughout the course of the illness and surgery the woman constantly evaluates her symptoms and experiences by determining what is normal and what is abnormal by comparing her present symptoms with her past experiences and with those of her friends. It is through this process that a woman establishes a frame of reference for the *boundaries of normality* before, during, and after a hysterectomy.

In this chapter the experiences of women who undergo a hysterectomy will be presented and the strategies that the informants in this study used to address and resolve their health problem will be examined.[1] Finally the ways in which these women maintained their sense of integrity about their bodies and their lives will be explored.

Establishing the Boundaries of Normality

The experiences of women who undergo a hysterectomy begin with the onset of symptoms. During this period the informants in this study implemented a number of strategies in an attempt to control, limit, and normalize these symptoms. In this investigation, *establishing the boundaries of normality* emerged as the basic psychological

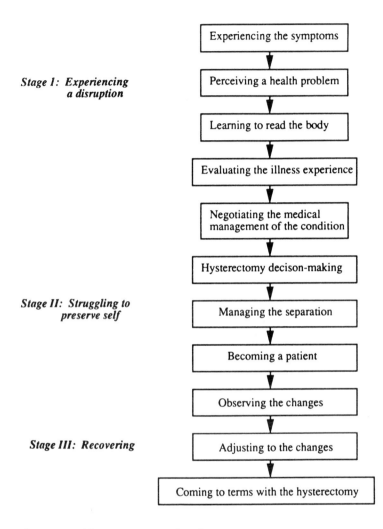

Figure 3.1. The Experience of Undergoing a Hysterectomy

process by which women coped with their symptoms and with the experience of a hysterectomy.

Establishing the boundaries of normality is defined as a process that involves incorporating what is unknown into that which is known, ordinary, and familiar. The women in this study sought to establish *boundaries of normality* by developing a frame of reference that helped explain their bodily changes. Through the process of establishing the boundaries of normality the informants attempted to understand their health problem, to remain in control of their bodily changes, and to protect their self-esteem (see Figure 3.2).

In order to understand their symptoms the informants reviewed their past menstrual experiences and consulted their friends. This process helped the informants construct a frame of reference that described the normal range of women's menstrual experiences. For example, these women would compare the amount of menstrual flow, the severity of cramping, or the degree of back pain with the severity of symptoms experienced in the past and with the experiences of their friends in order to determine if their current symptoms were "serious" or still within the normal range. This process enabled the informants to comprehend the fact that they did have a health problem, guided them in selecting and implementing coping strategies, and provided them with a baseline for identifying new symptoms.

The women in this study used this frame of reference to address and deny the false beliefs of others related to their health problem and to their impending hysterectomy. This normality framework allowed the informants to maintain as normal a life as possible and to protect their self-esteem:

> I think the one thing that everybody worries about is because so many times when you hear people say the woman's had a hysterectomy they associate that her personality, her mind is also going to be affected. "Oh, they've pulled everything out you know. She's going to be crying a lot; she won't understand." That seems to worry everybody because you're not just losing that womanly part of your body, you're afraid you're going to lose part of your marbles, part of your brain, and people are going to insinuate you can't reason well anymore because you had a hysterectomy. And I think that is why we are so concerned about being normal. I think I was . . . before I had this operation. . . . I didn't come about this operation . . . overnight, you know. I knew about it some time ago, so I had time to learn a lot and do some reading on it and know that most of the time that has nothing to do with your head, but a lot of people can't see that. . . . I think that's what worries us. Am I normal again now? Can I reason things out? Am I not going to burst out crying for anything?

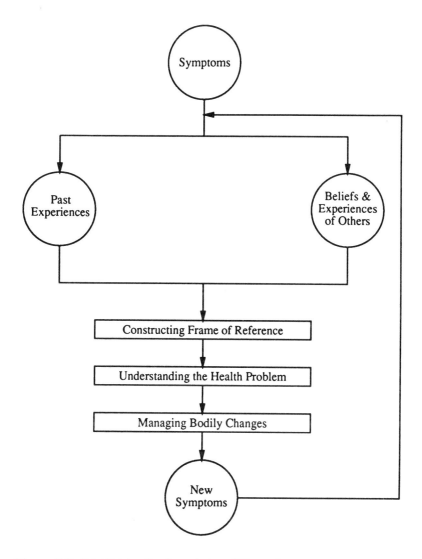

Figure 3.2. Establishing the Boundaries of Normality

The informants' *boundaries of normality* were repeatedly revised, however, as the health problem progressed and as new events and bodily changes occurred. The increasing severity of symptoms prompted the women to test and alter their frame of reference continuously by discussing aspects of their problem with others (including their husbands and physicians). This testing assisted them in maintaining their sense of competence about their changing situation; however, the informants were able to adjust their frame of reference only as long as others were willing to provide emotional and practical support.

Stage I: Experiencing a Disruption

Experiencing the Symptoms

Each woman who engaged in the process of preparing for, going through, and recovering from a hysterectomy did so in her own unique way. Although some variation existed in terms of their experiences with symptoms, however, there were also very definite patterns of behavior common to all members of the group.

The women's experiences with symptoms represent the first phase of the *Stage of Experiencing a Disruption*. Various combinations of eight major symptoms were outlined by informants: pain, bleeding, weakness, fatigue, shortness of breath, swelling, headaches, and lack of emotional control. Furthermore, the informants identified the symptoms of pain and bleeding as being central to their health problem. Time of occurrence, duration, frequency, and intensity of pain and bleeding were the most often discussed symptom characteristics. Figure 3.3 illustrates the variety of descriptors the women used to describe the symptoms of pain and bleeding.

All of the informants in this study said they were concerned about how their symptoms affected their life-style. The two most important aspects of their lives disrupted by the symptoms were sexuality and, for those who had not previously had a tubal ligation, birth control. The informants also said that the symptoms affected their performance on the job and their ability to function in the home.

Three of the five women in the study who had not had tubal ligations said they felt a great deal of anxiety regarding birth control while experiencing symptoms. These informants felt conventional methods of contraception such as the birth control pill were unreli-

Symptom Type	Time of Occurrence	Duration of Episode	Frequency	Intensity
• Pain	• Before / following ovulation • Before / following menstruation • Throughout cycle • During / following intercourse • During / following activities of daily living, ie. lifting, pushing, exercising • Following specific events, ie. vaginal exam, pap smear, laparoscopy, tubal ligation	• From a few minutes to 2 – 3 days	• From one to several times a day • Every day	• Very light • Aching • Sore • Sharp • Heavy and strong • Severe • Like labour
• Bleeding	• During / following ovulation • During menstruation • Throughout cycle • During / following intercourse • During / following activities of daily living, ie. lifting, pushing, exercising • Following specific events, ie. vaginal exam, tubal ligation	• From a few hours to several days	• From one to several times a day • Every day	• Spotting • Light • Moderate • Heavy • Saturating • With or without small to large clots

Figure 3.3. Descriptors of Pain and Bleeding

able because their body's natural rhythm was disrupted by the symptom episodes:

> I'd stay up until I made sure he was asleep or something, then I'd go to bed, or I'd sleep on the couch, not very often but, actually, quite a few times. You just get these silly ideas in your head. Don't touch me, I'll get pregnant. That's the way I was sometimes. I'd go like 42 days without a period and [think] oh God. Am I pregnant now? Then it [the bleeding] would come, bang, bang, bang. . . . I'd have to keep charts if I wanted to get pregnant and when I wanted to get pregnant.

The symptoms affected and disturbed these women's sexuality, and they experienced a decrease in their desire for intercourse because this exacerbated the symptoms. They were also concerned about feeling unattractive, about their partners' possible loss of interest in the relationship, and about the possibility of conceiving an unwanted or in some cases unaffordable child. One informant discussed this situation with her physician:

> I said, for the last four years, our sex life is the pits because it's getting to a point like for awhile there, well actually until now, for about three years straight I guess, sex wasn't interesting to me at all. I think it was probably because of my pains and what I was going through. I don't know, but I feel very sorry for my husband because he's been a very patient man. Most men wouldn't put up with something like that. They're usually used to having sex two or three times a week, and when it was getting to be like once or twice a month, you know, it's not fair to him either. And that was bothering me in the back of my mind. I told my physician, other than that we get along fine. I said, "My husband's been very patient. There are days when he has to have it, and you know, we make do somehow. Unfortunately, then I suffer for about three or four days." And I was telling him about that. And he said, "Well, what do you want to do?"

For the informants who were employed outside the home, coping with symptoms and maintaining energy often meant using sick days as one of the measures to establish symptom control. This was especially true for informants who held jobs that required a great deal of physical activity such as lifting, pushing, and pulling heavy objects. Those who went to work in spite of the severity of their symptoms found that their effectiveness and the quality of their performance suffered. They lacked stamina and felt exhausted most of the time. In addition adhering to strict work schedules made it difficult for these informants to control their symptoms:

> I started working a year and a half ago. That was one of the reasons this came to a head, too. When I was at home, I could cope because you can lay on the couch all day or whatever. . . . If things don't get done, it's not so bad; but at work, you know, you can't be expected to take it off all the time.

Those informants who worked on their own time and at their own pace had greater flexibility in terms of implementing coping strategies. As a result they were more successful in maintaining their energy and controlling symptoms than the women whose employment did not allow such flexibility.

The informants also said the symptoms affected their performance in the home. When symptom episodes were severe the women had difficulty fulfilling their role as mothers. Relinquishing household tasks to the husband or to an older child was very difficult for the informants in this study and they were frustrated when they did not have the strength or stamina to perform their usual activities. They became upset with implementing coping measures, which often involved sleeping after taking analgesics or postponing plans for family outings:

> It really got to me because I wouldn't know where [the symptoms would occur]. . . . I knew if I was driving somewhere and it happened, I couldn't drive; I would have to stop the vehicle.

Some of the informants said that their symptoms of pain and/or bleeding made them irritable and less tolerant of their family's demands. For others the lack of emotional control was identified as a symptom separate and apart from the pain and/or bleeding:

> You just get to a point where you're so tired, so tired all the time, you know. "Get these kids out of here!" You know, they just get on your nerves so much, and it was steady.

> I had mood swings so bad that one minute I'd be happy and the next minute I'd be tearing him apart or anybody else that stepped in my way. . . . Then I'd sit there and go "Holy but Jesus," you know, and then I'd go back to mellow again and just hateful, hateful moods. "Just get out of my sight. Don't talk to me, don't come near me. I'll kill anybody that comes near me." I thought, "Oh I can't handle this anymore." One minute I'm in a good mood, and then, for absolutely no reason, I'd turn into a complete animal. I'm surprised anybody still talks to me. I've snapped off more than a few heads.

Some of the informants attributed symptoms such as weakness, fatigue, shortness of breath, swelling, and headaches to their pain and bleeding. For example, these informants felt their weakness, fatigue, and shortness of breath were associated with their loss of blood. Other informants did not make this association and they felt these symptoms were separate entities.

Perceiving a Health Problem

Some of the informants lived with relatively severe symptoms for as long as ten years before becoming concerned enough to seek medical help and seriously consider having a hysterectomy. These informants realized they had a health problem when certain conditions in their lives changed. This health problem was ignored, however, as long as the following four symptom conditions remained unchanged: the symptoms were few in number; they were consistent and predictable; they were not perceived to alter one's life-style in unacceptable ways; and they could be justified as a normal occurrence in the female life cycle:

> I was a late bloomer, as they classify it, because I didn't start my period till I was fifteen years old; and from day one, I had severe cramps, a lot of very bad cramps, since I was a little girl, you know, fifteen. I was usually sick the first two days, right in bed with the cramps, and my mom always brought me up to believe that that was just part of life. And I went for so many years, and then when I had my first child everybody said, "Oh have a baby, and it will get easier." And with me, it went the exact opposite: It got worse.

The informants became concerned and anxious when symptom characteristics changed, when new symptoms appeared, when significant others began to consider their symptoms serious, when measures used to achieve symptom control demanded more time and energy, or when measures failed to produce the desired level of control. When any of these conditions occurred the informants began to suspect their symptoms indicated a problem with the uterus.

The perception of having a health problem represents the second phase of the *Stage of Experiencing a Disruption*. The realization that they were ill was the factor that forced the informants to explore their symptoms systematically in order to identify their *boundaries of normality*. Establishing these boundaries included assessing the characteristics, context and evolution of symptoms, as well as assessing and testing a variety of options for obtaining relief.

Learning to Read the Body

The informants in this study learned to *read their bodies* when they became concerned about their symptoms and recognized they were ill. *Learning to Read the Body* is the third phase of the *Stage of Experiencing a Disruption,* and it involves a set of specific activities systematically implemented by informants for the purpose of making sense of, coping with, and coming to terms with their health problem. The activities in this phase included evaluating symptoms and their characteristics, identifying and recognizing triggers of symptoms, assessing and testing options to find relief and the cause of the health problem, and seeking information and comparing symptoms with other women. These activities were instrumental in prolonging this particular phase because the consideration, testing, and evaluation of options often involved a "wait and see" period. In addition these activities tended to be repeated over and over again by the women in this study and the cyclical nature of these activities represents another factor that extended this phase.

When the informants initially began the phase of *Learning to Read the Body* they altered certain aspects of their lives in order to establish control over their symptoms and to assess whether these changes would shed light on the possible causes of their health problem. The informants' concerns about their bodies increased as their health problems intensified and as coping measures began to fail to relieve their symptoms. In order to manage their health problems successfully, the informants said they gradually involved significant others in managing their symptoms and making sense of the situation. The involvement of others often generated new options for finding relief as well as new ideas about the possible causes of their symptoms.

In addition to involving more and more individuals, the options considered and tested during this phase became more complex. The informants decided on which options to use after considering the effects these options would have on their bodies as well as on their family and job situations. Consuming a variety of over-the-counter analgesics represents one kind of option that produced changes in the informants' bodies as well as in their environment. Pain could be controlled or relieved by the ingestion of analgesics; however, drowsiness often resulted from this coping measure.

Over time and after having considered, tested, and evaluated a variety of options that yielded little relief and few answers the informants became "fed up" with having to plan their lives around their symptoms. They also became increasingly concerned about their limited success in managing their symptoms. In addition, significant others such as husbands were also affected by the informants' symptoms. For example, after a while some husbands feared that the illness was becoming quite serious and they urged their wives to consult a physician. Other husbands reacted differently: over time they became less tolerant of the effects of their wives' symptoms. The significant others' reactions to the informants' health problem and to their increasing inability to manage their symptoms were the two factors that motivated informants to seek assistance from health professionals.

When the informants consulted physicians they sought a label for their illness as well as some type of medical management for their health problem. As a result of consulting physicians these women were faced with a variety of medical options. Unlike previously tested coping measures these options often involved procedures that had to be carried out in the hospital and therefore were considered disruptive. Consenting to a laparoscopy illustrates this particular situation.

Individual differences influenced the length of time spent and the energy expended in attempting to read the body and discover the cause of the symptoms. These individual differences included the woman's knowledge of her body and her beliefs about that knowledge, her problem-solving and information-seeking behaviors, her tolerance to anxiety, pain, and bleeding, and her values and beliefs related to her symptoms and her uterus. In addition the major factors in this particular phase were differences in family, work, and relationship demands; the nature and quality of the woman's support system; the values and beliefs of significant others about the symptoms; and significant others' reactions to the symptoms and to the means used to achieve symptom control:

> He [the husband] was tired because I got very severe PMS [Premenstrual Syndrome] where I would literally throw things. I got almost an insane feeling about a week before my period, and I would break glasses, I would throw things. I was . . . the worse person. I could say other names for myself, but he couldn't really deal with that anymore. . . . I was like a time bomb ready to go off at any time when I had that.

The *Learning to Read the Body* phase contained specific patterns of behavior that were common to all the informants in this study (see Figure 3.4).

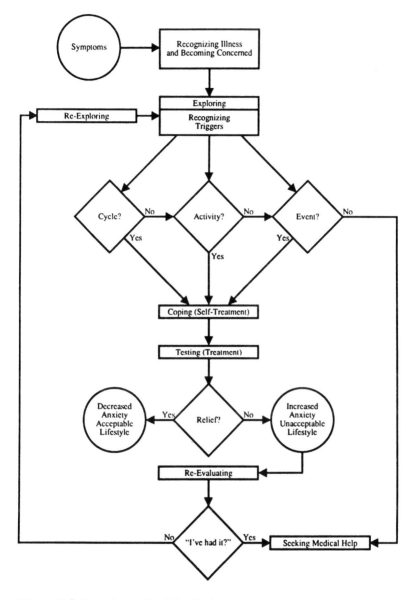

Figure 3.4. Learning to Read the Body

Exploring/Recognizing Triggers

When engaged in the *Learning to Read the Body* phase the informants first attempted to explore, by themselves and later with others,
a variety of factors that might trigger the onset of symptoms. Recognizing and controlling triggers helped the informants set limits to
their symptoms and three general categories of triggers were identified: the menstrual cycle, activities of daily living, and events occurring in their lives.

Cycle Triggers

When exploring symptom triggers the informants first examined
their symptoms in terms of their menstrual cycle in order to determine whether there was a relationship between symptom characteristics and specific stages of the cycle. The assessment of cycle triggers
was carried out over a period of several cycles in order to confirm
suspected relationships. In addition, exploring cycle triggers was the
starting point for all the informants in this phase because it was a
familiar aspect of their lives:

> That's why I was so surprised 'cause like the cramps over the years . . .
> had been really bad. I've tried all kinds of different drugs and stuff to get
> them under control, but over the last few years, it's really been bad. They
> always started about a week before. I couldn't do nothing the first few
> days into the period, but other than that, there was nothing out of the
> ordinary, nothing to pay any attention to.

Except when symptoms were extremely severe the examination
of cycle triggers was carried out with little or no interaction with
significant others. This initial questioning was focused specifically
on the body's natural rhythm and generally these questions did not
lead the informants to discuss their problem with others.

When the informants found a cycle trigger that was directly related
to their symptoms, they attempted to control the situation by testing a variety of self-treatment strategies, for example consuming a
variety of over-the-counter or prescription drugs, increasing rest
periods, and decreasing activities (such as intercourse and family
outings) at specific times during the cycle. When these strategies
brought relief, the informants felt less concerned about their bodies,

and they incorporated these measures into their life-style. On the other hand, when these strategies failed to relieve the symptoms the informants became anxious and they would then seek and test new options:

> I started out using Midol and aspirin and over-the-counter pain killers, but they didn't seem to help. Usually, I would go to bed with the electric blanket and turn it up full blast and drink tea. For some reason, tea seemed to help, and this would be for a day, usually the first day. And then, when I went on the pill, all of that stopped, and I had a very mild period.

Over time the strategies used to alleviate symptoms failed to control the health problem and the informants reevaluated their symptoms, comparing them with past experiences. They also began to discuss their symptoms with their husbands and to compare their problems with other women. These activities often led to new opinions, new ideas about the causes of their symptoms, and the discovery of new triggers. Finally, talking about their concerns with others provided the informants with some support and reassurance.

Activity Triggers

Activity triggers were considered when self-treatment strategies were no longer effective and when recognized cycle triggers no longer explained the onset of symptoms. In this case symptom characteristics were examined for any relationship with daily activities such as exercises, vacuuming, lifting, pushing, pulling, or intercourse:

> For at least ten years, I had pain on the right side, and that pain would vary depending on a lot of things, like my weight, how often sexual intercourse was being performed; and then also, it would have to do with my periods, and when I was really physically active.

When a relationship was recognized between symptom characteristics and specific activities the women tested new options such as decreasing the frequency of problem activities, relinquishing them to others, or ceasing them altogether. If relief was obtained, anxiety decreased and these additional measures were integrated into the informant's life-style. If there was no relief, the informants reevaluated their health problem with significant others and compared their symptoms with other women. Again, new options, new ideas about the cause of their symptoms, and new triggers often emerged from these exchanges.

Event Triggers

Event triggers, the final type of trigger, were examined when identified cycle and activity triggers no longer explained the onset of symptoms. In this case the informants explored their symptoms by looking for a relationship between the symptoms and specific events in their lives. The informants believed events such as giving birth, vaginal infections, a miscarriage, a tubal ligation, or stresses (such as looking for work or financial difficulties) were related to their symptoms:

> After I had my son, when I had my first period after, for no apparent reason, I'd get this sharp, stabbing pain right up inside of me. I was sitting here, and then all of a sudden, this stabbing pain would come up.

The informants in this study attempted to cope with their symptoms on their own when they identified a relationship between symptoms and a particular life event. In this case they watched the symptoms to assess whether the health problem decreased over time. When symptoms did not subside and when new symptoms appeared the informants experienced a great deal of concern about their bodies. Eventually the women realized they were no longer capable of managing their symptoms by themselves and they sought medical help in order to resolve their health problems.

Trigger Combinations

As their health problems became more complex and difficult to manage the informants said they consulted physicians and continued their attempts to read their bodies with others. Over time most of the informants identified a number of triggers related to their symptoms. A variety of trigger combinations were recognized and a number of self-treatment strategies which were more or less effective were developed to deal with the health problem. Gradually the informants' attempts to manage their symptoms created an unacceptable life-style, a life-style ruled by the informants' health problem:

> This started going on and on. The periods lasted longer, cramps were getting a lot worse; they started almost a week and a half before the period, going through all that. I went back to the doctor [to] see what I could get for it. I think he took another test, and everything was clear. One day, I started getting hostile with him. I was really getting frustrated. I started getting a lot of pain just by doing a little bit of pushing, and the next thing, if I lifted anything heavy, I'd get it. And always with the pain, I got bleeding, spotting, and the clots were really getting huge; and then, my period would stop; and then you figured you were all finished, and three or four days later, fluuushhh, one big clot, no warning, no nothing.

Only one informant did not engage to any great extent in testing self-treatment strategies in the *Learning to Read the Body* phase. In this instance the informant failed to identify any triggers for her symptoms. Furthermore, she was not only concerned and anxious about her illness but she was afraid of cancer because she had been treated a number of years earlier for cancer of the cervix. Unlike the other nine informants this woman immediately sought medical assistance for managing her health problem, and her particular pattern of behavior is represented in Figure 3.4 by the lateral pathway between each type of trigger:

> It was nothing that was definite. You couldn't put a finger on when you were going to get it. Like it had nothing to do with the menstrual cycle at all, nothing. Like, I don't know how to explain it. I could be sitting or standing or something and just get these sharp pains.

Evaluation of the Illness Experience

The outcome of the informants' interactions with others directly affected how they viewed and coped with their illness during the *Learning to Read the Body* phase. Husbands, significant women such as mothers or close female friends, and physicians were the types of people whom the informants approached for help with their health problem.

The informants sought to measure the impact of their health problem on their husbands and on the family as a whole when they talked about their symptoms with their spouses. They also attempted to obtain their families' support and assistance with tasks in the home. The husbands' abilities to recognize, support, and discuss the health problem varied greatly in this study. Several of the informants said their husbands recognized and were willing to discuss their health problem. Some of these husbands actively supported their wives with tasks in the home, although others provided limited assistance in this area.

One of the women in this study was divorced and became involved in another relationship during the *Stage of Experiencing a Disruption*. The involvement of this partner was less intense in the process than the involvement of the other informants' husbands. In this instance the woman identified her mother as the individual who assisted and supported her the most during her illness.

Some of the informants said their husbands had difficulty recognizing the existence of their illness and were not open to discussing the issues surrounding their health problem. These informants also said they received no emotional or functional support from their husbands; consequently, they had difficulty accurately measuring the impact of their health problem on their marriage:

> It was very trying on the relationship I'll tell you. . . . You don't know if he's lost interest or something like that or something to that effect.

When the informants approached the significant women in their lives they were able to freely discuss most issues surrounding their health problem. These individuals quickly recognized the illness and they displayed greater empathy than the husbands because many of them had experienced this type of health problem and, therefore, had a good understanding of its impact on the informant and on her marital and familial relationships. In many instances significant women were valuable sources of information and support because they could explain the symptoms, provide reassurance, and suggest new options for finding relief:

> I tried these different kinds of herbs and things. My aunt sent away somewhere and got me those. I was on those for a month or more. . . . It was my aunt who told me that these were mixed with vitamins and stuff, and they were suppose to be high, really high in vitamins and everything; and she was on them, and [I] thought, well, might as well try them.

Some of the informants had problems finding significant women from whom to obtain support and assistance. For example, one woman in this study had little contact with the significant women in her life. In this instance her mother and sisters did not live in the same country and she had few close female friends residing in the city. She said this situation made it difficult for her to cope with and understand her health problem: "I felt lonely, alone, not knowing what's happening and what's not happening, you know."

The recognition of the health problem by the spouse and the accessibility of significant women emerged as two important factors influencing the way women in this study viewed and coped with their illness during the *Learning to Read the Body* phase. The outcomes resulting from the presence or the absence of one or both of these factors are described and examined below and illustrated in Figure 3.5.

The informants were able to adjust to their illness when their husbands recognized their health problems and when there were significant women to provide emotional support and information (Figure 3.5, Cell *a*). In this instance the informants said they were supported and assisted by their husbands, which made it possible for them to implement a variety of coping measures designed to relieve their symptoms. They also said the information provided by significant women helped them to develop an *explanatory model* for their illness. The notion of an explanatory model refers to the ways in which the informants articulated and discussed their symptoms. Having an explanatory model helped the informants make the illness experience clear to others and it allowed them to expand their repertoire of coping strategies as they progressed through the *Stage of Experiencing a Disruption*. As a result these particular women managed their illness for a long period of time before seeking medical assistance.

Other informants said they felt isolated when they could not find significant women who could provide support and information (Figure 3.5, Cell *b*). Although their husbands recognized the existence of their health problem, these particular women had no references for comparing symptoms and as a result they felt limited in their ability to cope. They had difficulty developing an explanatory model for their illness and they could not expand their repertoire of coping strategies during the *Learning to Read the Body* phase because opportunities for discussing their concerns with significant women

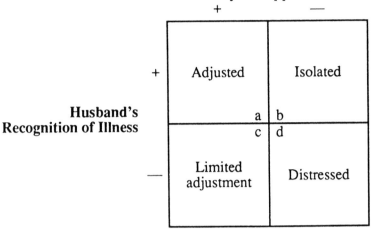

Figure 3.5. Influence of Significant Others on Women's Coping

were few or nonexistent. Consequently these informants tended to seek medical assistance in order to manage and understand their condition very early in their illness.

Some of the informants felt limited in their ability to adjust to their illness because their husbands did not recognize their health problem (Figure 3.5, Cell *c*). Although these informants did not receive support from their husbands, they did have access to information from significant women which helped them develop an explanatory model for their health problem. Women significant to the informants also suggested a variety of coping measures for relieving symptoms; however, these informants often could not implement particular coping strategies, such as reducing the frequency of intercourse or relinquishing tasks to others, because their husbands viewed these measures as disruptive and unwarranted. These particular informants said they attempted to cope as best they could but they eventually sought medical assistance as the health problem became more acute and the strain on their marital relationship increased.

The informants felt distressed about their illness when their husbands did not recognize their health problem and when there were no available significant women with whom to discuss their symptoms (Figure 3.5, Cell *d*). In these cases the informants were very concerned about their health problem and became afraid as they failed to make sense of it. They were limited in their attempts to cope during the *Learning to Read the Body* phase because their husbands did not tolerate their coping measures and their repertoire of strategies to manage symptoms was poor. Like the informants who had little access to significant women (Figure 3.5, Cell *b*), these informants sought medical assistance early in their illness.

As the informants progressed through the *Stage of Experiencing a Disruption* certain events were identified which improved or impeded the women's ability to cope, and these events changed the informants' perception of their illness. The events included the provision of medical information that confirmed the illness to their husbands, the gradual loss of emotional and functional support from spouses as they became tired of dealing with their wives' illness, an increased accessibility to significant women, and a decreased accessibility to significant women.

Consulting a physician was a coping strategy implemented during the *Learning to Read the Body* phase. The informants selected and tested this particular coping strategy when they were unable to manage their symptoms appropriately and when they received positive or negative cues from their husbands and significant women. For example, husbands who expressed their concerns about the illness and urged their wives to see a doctor illustrate a positive cue. In contrast, husbands who did not recognize or were unconvinced of the existence of the health problem represent a negative cue. In the instance of a negative cue the informants felt that consulting a doctor was the only way they could convince their husbands they were ill.

When the informants consulted physicians they were seeking confirmation, a label, and a medical solution for their health problem. They wanted to identify the cause of their problem and obtain expert advice on how to manage and resolve the symptoms. Although the informants' success in addressing these issues with their physicians varied greatly, a few informants were successful in their initial interactions with their doctors. In these instances the informants said their physicians were empathetic and acknowledged their illness:

Yeah, he let me read the report from the laparoscopy, which, like I said, I don't know of any other doctor that would let you read the report and then sit down and explain it to you.

I went to a doctor that really straightened everything out. He was a very patient, very good doctor. He would really listen, and his diagnosis was very good on a great many things, and he actually educated us more than any doctor we've ever known. He's the one who explained that things were not really critical but that it would not really get better. And he explained to me . . . when things did get kind of bad just before that last child was born that he thought it was better for me to have a hysterectomy. . . . We told him no, and he understood, and he said that he would try and help us, you know, as long as my health was still doing all right, he would help us as much as possible.

The majority of the informants, however, had little or no success in their initial encounters with physicians. In these instances the physicians did not address the concerns of the women. These consultations frustrated the informants because their doctors did not acknowledge the impact of the illness on their lives; consequently these women went from one doctor to the next until they found one who verified their health problem and responded to their concerns with empathy and respect:

We left that doctor's office because he was very rude and insinuated that all of this was my husband's fault. You know, something about didn't we know anything about birth control? Didn't he realize how bad my health was? We just got up and left.

The problem started after my son was born, about when I went back for my six weeks check-up, and she just said it was probably because I had just had a baby and give it time; and I never really paid attention to it, but then I started getting my menstruations every week, so I kept going back to her. At first she thought it was a growth inside. It can go on in the womb, or it can go on anywhere. So they did an exploratory on me, and they found out that wasn't it. So then she said, "Well, there's really nothing they could do. Just carry on and ignore it." . . . She just kept saying "It's in your head" or "Don't worry about it." She said, "We could do a hysterectomy, but I don't think that's your problem. I think it's just you know you." So I decided to go for a second opinion.

As the informants progressed through the *Stage of Experiencing a Disruption* most of them became increasingly affected by their husbands' and physicians' reactions. Husbands became either very concerned about their wives or very intolerant of the effects of their symptoms and coping measures. Furthermore, in spite of the fact that the informants continued to interact with other women they also realized that the lay management of their illness was insufficient to address their health problem effectively. Consequently the informants increasingly began to rely on their physicians to manage their condition medically.

The acknowledgment of their health problem by a physician and the recognition of their illness by their husband were two factors that influenced the way informants coped and viewed their illness during the later period of the *Stage of Experiencing a Disruption*. The outcomes resulting from the presence or the absence of one or both of these factors are explained below and summarized in Figure 3.6.

The informants were able to confirm and label their health problem successfully when their physicians acknowledged their illness and when their husbands provided emotional and functional support (Figure 3.6, Cell *a*). Informants in this situation tested a variety of medical options and felt supported by their husbands who often assumed household tasks when these women were unable to carry out their normal activities.

When husbands did not recognize the illness in the later period of the *Stage of Experiencing a Disruption* it became a priority for the informants to convince their husbands of their condition because their symptoms were becoming more acute and increasingly difficult to manage (Figure 3.6, Cell *c*). Although their physicians confirmed their illness, these women found the medical management of their condition difficult as their husbands did not support the implementation and testing of various medical options. Therefore, in order to obtain support and relieve the strain on their marital relationship, these informants often used data from diagnostic tests to convince their husbands of their illness.

When physicians failed to acknowledge their illness the informants became frustrated and they searched for a doctor who would listen and respond to their concerns (Figure 3.6, Cell *b*). In this instance the husbands supported their wives and often assisted them in their attempts to find appropriate medical assistance.

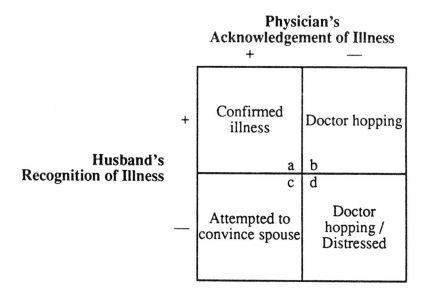

Figure 3.6. Influence of Spouse and Physicians on Women's Coping and View of Illness

The failure to locate a doctor who would acknowledge their health problem overwhelmed the informants when their husbands did not recognize their illness (Figure 3.6, Cell *d*). In these cases symptoms were becoming increasingly difficult to manage and the informants had few means available to convince their husbands of their illness. These informants searched for a physician on their own and they said this situation was stressful.

Negotiating the Medical Management of the Condition

As the *Stage of Experiencing a Disruption* progressed the informants became increasingly involved in the *medical management of their condition* and they felt this form of management was different from the lay illness management provided by significant women. Most of the informants felt apprehensive during their encounters with doctors because they thought physicians were powerful and possessed expert and privileged information about the human body. In addition the informants were aware that doctors control access to potent medications and a variety of diagnostic and treatment procedures. The perception of physicians as powerful created situations in which most of the informants felt disadvantaged when attempting to find the cause of and relief from their health problem. A few of the informants felt confident about their understanding of the medical jargon and the medical care system, and these informants were assertive during their consultations with doctors. Most of the informants, however, often acquiesced to their physicians' suggestions with little or no negotiation as they had difficulty assessing whether an option was appropriate or not:

> So I told him I wanted a D & C [dilatation and curettage]. Maybe that will do it. He goes, "Well, sometimes it helps, sometimes it don't." He said, "But if you really want to take that route first and see if it helps, then we'll try it."

> I went to the doctor, and she asked me all these personal questions about how you get along with your husband and all this stuff, and I said fine. I said other than sometimes we think about our finances, but that's normal in this day and age, everything else seems to be just fine. I'm working, my husband's working, no problems. So she checked me and everything, and she asked me where the pains were. So she started giving me antibiotics. She thought maybe it was an infection of some sort. So she gave me antibiotics, and the pain subsided for awhile, and then they came back again. And I kept going to Dr. ____, and every time I would be going back to her, she would be giving some other medication. Then she told me, "The only way that we're going to find out what's wrong in there is if you go for an ultrasound." So I went for an ultrasound.

Over time physicians and informants implemented, tested, and exhausted a number of medical options for diagnosing and controlling the health problem. In some instances the informants felt secure about the medical management of their illness and they thought a trusting relationship had been established with their doctors. In other cases the informants felt less secure about the medical management of their condition. These informants said they did not know their doctors very well and they were reluctant to express many of their concerns:

> Well, sometimes when you don't really know the doctor that well you're kind of nervous to ask all the personal questions. It's a little different if he's your family doctor and you've known him for years and you can joke around with him and whatever, like a normal person. Someone that you only see maybe once every two to three years or whatever. . . . it's not someone that you can get really close to.

Because the informants continued to suffer symptoms, medical options became increasingly complex because more intrusive procedures were being used to manage the symptoms and to diagnose the health problem precisely. Procedures such as a dilatation and curettage or a laparoscopy are examples of these intrusive procedures. Following these procedures some of the informants were informed that abnormalities such as fibroids or adhesions had been identified and were probably related to their symptoms. In other cases, however, no abnormalities were found and as a result these women often began to worry that an undiscovered malignancy might be the underlying cause of their health problem.

After testing these particular diagnostic and treatment measures physicians began to discuss the option of having a hysterectomy. Unlike the previously tested surgical options this form of surgical management did not allow for testing as it was irreversible. The informants reacted in a variety of ways to this option. Some of them felt shock and disbelief, while others felt overwhelmed by the irreversible nature of this surgery:

> He said, "There might be a few fibroids there. Sooner or later, it could be a year, it could be two, three, or whatever," he said, "but you're a candidate for a hysterectomy sooner or later." [I said], "What, are you crazy? I'm too young for that ain't I?" 'Cause to me, I always thought a hysterectomy . . . meant you had to go on these change of life and all that other stupid stuff. But then again, I was in pain off and on all the time, but I could still handle it.

The issue of having a hysterectomy was presented to the women in this study as the final option for resolving their health problem. The informants were informed by their physicians that a hysterectomy would mean removing the uterus and one or both ovaries if they were damaged. Most doctors explained that they would attempt to preserve one or both ovaries because this would prevent the onset of menopause. One of the informants said that she did not understand the meaning of preserving or removing ovaries and that her doctor had been unclear about this issue:

> See, I really didn't understand a whole lot about it. I mean, I knew what I had to know about it, but as far as having one ovary and taking one, I would have just as soon they took them both. I don't know.

All of the informants were told that this surgery would probably alleviate their symptoms and that a hysterectomy would not negatively affect their sexual activities. The informants said that the physicians were very explicit about the fact that except for this surgery they could offer no other form of treatment to manage their condition appropriately:

> "Well," he said, "there really is no alternative." He said, "There's no pill or anything to correct this. You know, we don't do this just to anybody. A hysterectomy is serious, so you should really think about it."

The Hysterectomy Decision-Making Process

There was considerable variation in the way the informants in this study made their decision to have a hysterectomy. One informant said her physician and her husband made the decision for surgery. In this instance the doctor scheduled the surgery and did not give her time to make a decision. She discussed the issue with her husband on the following day and she said that he responded rationally and objectively to the situation. He weighed the pros and cons of having a hysterectomy and he quickly concluded that the surgery was the best option. This woman added that her husband did not consider her feelings and concerns about this alternative and she felt distressed by his lack of attention to her emotional needs:

> You know, it was like good points, bad points, stick it together and see what are the advantages and disadvantages of it and then decide on it. . . . I was nervous. I was worried. What about after the surgery? The pain or whatever goes with it for six weeks, and [it eliminates] having any more kids.

One informant decided on her own to have the hysterectomy. In this instance her boyfriend and mother were excluded from the decision-making process. She said that her doctor was very support-ive and that she had a great deal of trust in his expertise. When the option was presented she discussed her concerns with her physician and immediately agreed to have the hysterectomy. She felt confident about her choice and she said she had a thorough understanding of the situation. Furthermore, she knew about the implications of this surgery because her mother had experienced it a number of years earlier:

> Well, I had already made the decision. I had decided even before I left the doctor's office. I told him, "Yes, we will go ahead and do this because I don't want to go through the pain." And you know, it was getting to look like I was pregnant again with the swelling.

Some of the informants made their decision for surgery jointly with their husbands. In these instances the physicians presented the option but did not participate in the decision-making process. These informants waited as long as several months before making their decision and they used this time to consider the implications of having or not having the surgery.

The hysterectomy decision-making process was considered very painful by one informant and her husband. Although they both agreed that living with the symptoms was unacceptable, they had difficulty coming to terms with the fact that the surgery would mean abandoning their plan to have one more child:

> My son is two now. He's not really a baby anymore. He's growing up on us. And we sit back and we think, I don't remember him as a baby, and that took a lot out of him [the husband]. He said, "You know, if things would have worked out, I would have liked another child." He didn't help the situation because he had the baby bug, too.

Some of the informants decided to have the surgery when they realized that they could no longer cope with their symptoms. Unfor-tunately the spouses of these women expressed their opposition to the option because they worried that the hysterectomy would affect their wives sexually or that they might die from the surgery. These informants eventually convinced their husbands that it was neces-sary to have the surgery:

He wasn't keen on the idea when I first told him about it back in November. He said, "No way, you're not going in for this surgery and so and so died from that. . . ." At the end, I had all kinds of thoughts. I even said to my husband a couple of times, "You know, something's growing in there, and I probably have a tumor the size of a football." He didn't take lightly to that comment.

One informant, who felt threatened by the hysterectomy option, consulted other physicians in order to confirm that this surgery was necessary to resolve her health problem. She had difficulty coming to terms with the idea of losing a part of her body. When she discussed the hysterectomy with her husband he immediately agreed to it because he was tired of dealing with her illness. He did not respond to her fears and concerns, and eventually he insisted she have the surgery. Consequently this woman felt that she had little input in the decision to have the hysterectomy. She coped with her feelings and her husband's lack of support by postponing the surgery until she felt ready to face it:

He didn't know about me canceling out. . . . I sort of made excuses 'cause he would phone and he would say, "Well did they call you today?" "No." I wasn't going to let him know . . . because he'd give me heck for it. But it was me that was going in, not him, and he would say, "Oh for God's sake, it's just an operation." Yeah right, you go in and have it for me then.

Other informants made the decision for surgery with the help of their husbands and physicians. In these instances the husbands were open to discussing the surgery but they recognized that their wives should make the final decision because the health problem and its resolution affected them the most. The physicians provided assistance by clarifying issues with the informants and their husbands. Consequently these women felt supported and they believed that their input in the decision-making process was important. One woman in this group postponed her decision to have a hysterectomy in order to have one more child. Most of these informants, however, chose to have the hysterectomy after deciding that they definitely did not want any more children:

Well he [the husband] said, "It's entirely up to you. If you don't want it, don't have it, but look at what you're living with now." He basically let me make my own mind up, and he said, "Whatever you decide that's fine." He felt that I should have it, but he said, "If you don't want it, you know, it's you going through it not me." No, he was quite supportive.

One informant let her doctor make the decision about the hysterectomy. She acquiesced because she was worried that a malignancy might be the underlying cause of her health problem. She had reservations about the surgery but she felt that she would be at risk if she refused to have it. In this instance the husband was excluded from the decision-making process. Although the husband supported the physician's decision, he did not respond to his wife's fears and concerns:

> It was under the understanding that whatever they found, they took it out rather than wake me up and say we got to do this and cut me open again. . . . [My husband said,] "If it was going to make everything better, then go for it." Whether I ever went back to work or whatever, like, he didn't care. He just wanted the problem fixed.

Stage II: Struggling to Preserve Wholeness

Managing the Separation

The informants' preparation for admission to the hospital marks the beginning of the second stage of the hysterectomy process: *Struggling to Preserve Wholeness*. At this point the informants in this study tried to minimize the effects their imminent departure from the home would have on their husbands and children. The informants made arrangements with extended family members or close friends to provide support and assistance for their family during their absence and a few of the informants enlisted the services of homemakers from a community agency. For some of the informants managing their separation from the family also included implementing additional measures such as assigning specific tasks to older children, preparing and freezing meals, and, most importantly, providing emotional support to their children by explaining to them the reasons for the hospitalization. The informants said they implemented these particular strategies so that their family's life would remain as normal as possible.

In addition the informants provided emotional and practical support for their husbands in order to preserve the integrity of their marital relationship. Most of the informants requested their husband's help in planning their departure from the home. By involving their husbands these women were able to clarify various aspects of family routines such as their children's extracurricular activities. Furthermore, during these exchanges the informants were able to assess the impact of their absence on their husbands' coping abilities. Several of the informants said that their husbands were very concerned about their ability to manage the family on their own. In these instances the informants had to reassure their husbands, for example they would remind their husbands that their stay in the hospital would be no longer than five or six days.

The informants had to manage their separation from the family throughout their hospitalization. They provided emotional support for their children by telephoning them as often as possible, although husbands were supported mostly when they visited their wives in hospital:

> I was separated from her [the oldest child] for six weeks when I was in there for my second one. I was on bed rest, and she thought I was going to be gone that long again. But I assured her not, four sleeps and one day, you know. So she marked each day off on a calendar, and then I talked to her on the phone quite a few times so it wasn't like I was totally not around.

> I wasn't there with him, and I wasn't there with the kids. . . . As soon as he'd get to the hospital, that's the first thing he'd say, "I can't even sleep nights 'cause you're not there." He'd say, "Well, what are the kids going to do, this and this is coming up, and you're not there." I'd say, "Well, mom is there, she's going to be able to take care. . . ." Then, when he'd get ready to leave, he'd say the same thing, "I just hate to leave you." I'd go, "Well honey, you've got to go home and go to bed, you know. . . ." That separation did seem to have played a very big part with him and the kids. It did.

Becoming a Patient

The informants assumed the patient role when they were admitted to the hospital. For most of the informants the patient role was disturbing and difficult. When they described their experiences as patients the women focused on two particular aspects: their lack of control and their sense of fragmentation. The informants described lack of control in terms of their limited opportunities to initiate, select, and orchestrate events. Because the hospital was an unfamiliar setting most of the informants felt uncomfortable making requests; consequently they experienced a loss of control over the situation. For example, this lack of control occurred when the women were unable to manage certain self-care activities such as pain control:

> It's frustrating when they give you something for pain, and it doesn't take the pain away. You can't have anything for four hours. At home, I just take some more Tylenol.

The informants said they felt a sense of fragmentation because the health professionals concentrated on their illness and organs and ignored them as individuals. Their sense of fragmentation was evident in their descriptions of various hospital procedures: for example, they said the health professionals focused on specific body parts and functions or on specific tasks (e.g., taking a history) without recognizing them as individuals or attending to all of their needs, both physical and emotional:

> When the intern came in to take a history, I told him, "I don't know what's wrong." I said, "Could you please ask him [the gynecologist] if he can do a tubal instead. . . ." He said, "He would do a hysterectomy because I wasn't planning any more kids. . . ." I just didn't know anything about the side-effects or what happens once you have this done, so I was worried, you know. . . . They were preparing me for the surgery but not with the information about what it is.

> At one point . . . an intern [came] in, and she kept asking me these questions about breast cancer and stuff like that and looking at me like I was nuts. And then she said, "Well, you're in here to get a lump removed from your breast aren't you?" And I said, "No." I didn't need to hear that. . . . She said, "Well, we must have you mixed up," and I thought, "You do the right operation."

Although the informants assumed and viewed the patient role in different ways, these variations depended on two factors: the informants' knowledge of hospital rituals and their mastery of medical language. In this context the term *ritual* comprises procedures that served to prepare the informants for the surgical event as well as the routine nursing care interventions carried out during the postoperative period. Being examined by health professionals, receiving information about the surgery and its immediate effects, and giving formal consent for the hysterectomy are examples of hospital rituals. In contrast, the concept of *mastery* relates to the informants' understanding of medical terminology and their ability to use medical terms. The outcomes resulting from the presence or the absence of one or both of these factors are described below and summarized in Figure 3.7.

The patient role was described positively when the informants understood the medical language and the purpose of various hospital rituals (Figure 3.7, Cell *a*). Only one informant in this study described her patient experience in positive ways. In this instance the informant said she felt in control and that she collaborated willingly with the hospital staff. She added that prior to her hospitalization her physician had been very thorough in explaining what would happen during and after the surgery. She said that he often clarified and defined the medical terms used to describe procedures, body parts and functions, and specific events that occur in the hospital. Consequently, she asked few questions while in the hospital because most of her concerns had been dealt with before her admission. Furthermore, this woman had been admitted to the same hospital unit a few months prior to her admission for the hysterectomy. She remembered and knew the rituals and she said that the staff members remembered her. She felt that the health professionals were concerned about the well-being of her whole person and therefore she experienced no sense of fragmentation:

> The staff there were excellent. The nurses were excellent, you know, the doctor and his staff. . . . That was the ward I was on six months ago, so I already knew all the nurses and most of them remembered me. . . . You know, I felt like I was at home.

Most of the informants in this study said they found the patient role uncomfortable or disturbing. Some of these informants understood the medical language, but they were unclear about the underlying purpose of specific hospital rituals (Figure 3.7, Cell *c*). For other women, however, the situation was different: They did not understand the medical terminology but they knew and understood most

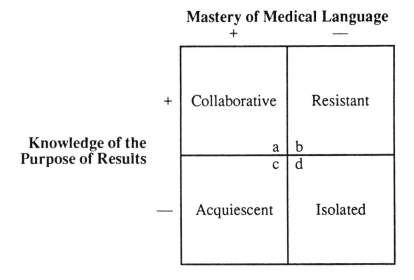

Figure 3.7. Women's Perceptions of the Patient Role

of the hospital rituals (Figure 3.7, Cell *b*). In both instances these informants felt they were partially in control of events because they understood either some of the medical language or the purpose of most of the hospital rituals. They tended to feel confident about their knowledge and they asked health professionals questions in an attempt to deal with their concerns.

Although the factors were different, both groups of women experienced a sense of fragmentation during hospital procedures. Those who mastered the medical language described their fragmentation in terms of feeling ill at ease with rituals they felt were demeaning (Figure 3.7, Cell *c*). Furthermore, as these particular informants relied on health professionals to guide them through hospital rituals they were careful not to jeopardize their relationships with them. Consequently, they often acquiesced to staff requests and refrained from complaining about procedures they disliked:

> I understand that years ago the procedures were that there always had to be a woman nurse present, and now it depends on the doctor. . . . I still

think, you know, even if you were to ask me I probably would be so embarrassed that I wouldn't say, "Yes, I want a female nurse present. . . ." I think they should have a nurse there period, all the time, and you could state it before you go in on a sheet or something so you don't have to be confronted with the doctor or feel that you're embarrassing him or hurting his feelings or something.

One informant experienced a sense of fragmentation when she signed the consent form for the operation because she discovered that another physician was consulted about the decision for her hysterectomy. Obtaining the opinion of two physicians before performing a hysterectomy is a requirement in Canadian hospitals for all women under 40 years of age. This informant felt this practice was particularly demeaning because it implied that she was "too young" to have the hysterectomy and therefore that she was unable to make a sound decision regarding the management of her health problem:

And I had to sign that form because I was too young for the surgery and all these things I had to do. It was like I just didn't understand anymore, like you had to have another doctor's signature because I was under 40, and I really felt like, God, I'm 12 years old, like, I'm not suppose to be having this surgery. It was very hard. I just felt like everybody was looking at me like this little girl is in for this surgery that she's too young for. You kind of got that impression, and I felt the nurses did. They babied me almost.

In contrast, those informants who knew and understood the hospital rituals and their purposes experienced a sense of fragmentation when health professionals used terminology they did not understand or when staff members failed to respond to their needs (Figure 3.7, Cell *b*). Unlike the informants who did not express their dislike of certain hospital rituals these informants attempted to resist those hospital rituals that they disliked and they often discussed these particular rituals with staff members and requested certain changes:

The morphine did nothing for me. It made me wide awake, and I told them three or four times. You know, you'd finally fall asleep and you'd feel another needle going into you. They didn't even ask you, so finally I said, "No more, give me a 292 or something." That I wasn't impressed with, the way they push drugs on you, take it, keep taking it, you know, it will make you feel better. It didn't help me at all. I was really turned off with that.

Some of the informants said they had a negative patient experience. For instance these informants had difficulty understanding the medical terminology as well as the purpose of most of the hospital rituals (Figure 3.7, Cell *d*). They felt they had no control over the events in the hospital and they experienced an acute sense of fragmentation. They were reluctant and embarrassed to clarify issues with health professionals because they were unsure about the questions they could or should ask as well as how and when to ask them. They acquiesced to requests from health professionals and coped with their feelings by limiting or avoiding interactions with the staff as much as possible:

Nobody told me anything. They would just come in and give me a shot for the pain and that's it. Nobody talked about anything. . . . I felt like I shouldn't be there. . . . I would feel hesitant to push the buzzer. After the second day, I felt like I shouldn't push the buzzer unless I really, really needed it.

They asked me to sign some forms, and I didn't know what that meant. They didn't answer me, tell me anything unless I asked them. And I'm shy, to a point, and I didn't know what to ask them. I didn't know what to expect or anything, so I didn't know what to ask them. . . . They use such big words and medical terms.

I was scared. I don't like to be alone, but I got a private room. I just didn't want to see anybody else, if that makes sense.

Some of the informants felt it was unreasonable and unwarranted for physicians who wanted to conduct a physical examination or for nurses who wanted to perform interventions such as giving an injection for pain or changing a dressing to ask their husbands to leave the room, and this practice increased their feeling of isolation. They said that this practice prevented them from receiving support and that it limited their attempts to manage their separation from their husbands:

They were several young male doctors that came in to examine me, and each time my husband was there, they would ask him to leave. And I did not know this till later, but that annoyed my husband very, very badly. . . . And you know, since then there's been a few comments from some of his friends, and it seems like most of the men would have felt the same way. They don't like the fact, you know, when it comes to that part, there just seems to be such a bond in there between a husband and a wife. It's almost like amputating part of you when you do that. Even though there's nothing physically happening to the husband, it affects him. If they're not let in on how to help you feel better, you feel like you can't get well because you have that problem of how am I going to make him understand. So that was very annoying.

During the hours preceding the hysterectomy the informants thought about their surgery and focused on one or more of the following four aspects: the body's reaction to the anaesthesia, how health professionals would handle their body, the possible discovery of cancer, and what would be removed and what would be left intact inside their body. They also considered some of the possible long-term effects of the surgery. These long-term effects included mental, emotional, and sexual changes, hormonal instability, and changes in their relationships with others:

> I was worried of literally dying, but I was also afraid that they might find cancer, and I was also concerned about my ovary and tube and how they would handle the hormonal imbalance. I was afraid of how I would react, whether there would be a mental change. Would I be really nervous or yelling or screaming or all these things that you hear? And I was also concerned about how this would affect a married life sexually.

The informants said they experienced sudden, severe physical symptoms such as pain, nausea, and vomiting immediately following the hysterectomy. They said they reacted to the intensity of their symptoms by focusing on their bodies. As a result their ability to cope with the outside world decreased and they required assistance from significant others and health professionals to carry out simple activities such as sitting at the bedside. Although all of the informants expected the occurrence of most symptoms, the feeling of being extremely vulnerable was an unforeseen emotional component of their hysterectomy experience.

The pain killers the informants received in the hospital intensified their feelings of vulnerability and loss of control. These substances changed the natural rhythm of the body by creating disturbances such as altered sleep patterns. In addition, the informants said these substances altered and impeded their ability to perceive and interpret reality. The informants attempted to minimize these side-effects as much as possible because they prevented them from accurately assessing their bodies and their environment.

Some of the informants tolerated the side-effects because they realized that the use of pain killers would decrease over time. In contrast, other informants attempted to moderate side-effects by requesting that intramuscular pain killers be discontinued and substituted by less potent medications. In these cases the informants said they felt it was easier to cope with the pain than to cope with the side-effects:

> I'm very confused about what happened there. When you're in a hospital, they have you so doped up that you don't think of asking the doctor different questions when you see him. On Saturday, I finally just asked them, I just told them, "Don't give me any more Demerol" because I just felt like I wasn't thinking anymore. I don't like the out of control feeling, so they were very nice that way, [and] they took me off of it. I was still in pain, but I thought I could deal with that a lot easier.

The informants felt reluctant to discuss the pain killers' side-effects with health professionals. For example, one woman said that morphine affected her sleep pattern, producing nightmares in which she experienced the sensation of falling. After one particularly unpleasant nightmare she told a nurse she needed to be held because she was afraid. In this instance the nurse did not acknowledge her distress or attempt to reassure her in any way. This informant was embarrassed by the disclosure of her feelings and was confused and angered by the nurse's reactions. She added that she did not attempt to talk about her feelings again.

Informants reported that the medication side-effects affected their ability to understand information. For example, physicians most often provided information about the surgery during the first days following the hysterectomy, the time when the side-effects were most acute. Consequently the informants said they had difficulty making sense of what was being explained to them and had to clarify this information when the side-effects had subsided:

What I didn't like was that when I first came out of surgery. . . . I remember him [the Doctor] vaguely telling me what kind of took place, and I expected him to come and retell me and explain to me, and he didn't. As a matter of fact, if I hadn't asked, I think maybe two days later, I wouldn't have really known, and that bothered me because I really wanted to know what happened, what was done to my body.

All of the informants openly discussed physical symptoms with health professionals. This was the strategy the informants used to understand what was happening inside their bodies. They said that the health professionals were supportive and supplied information about the frequency and cause of particular symptoms. For example, the nurses told some of the informants that the feeling "your insides were going to fall out" when standing up was in fact a normal, common sensation during the first few days following a hysterectomy, and they reassured the informants that this feeling would gradually subside.

Uncontrolled bleeding and bladder infections were the two most frequent complications reported by the informants. Some of the informants said they experienced uncontrolled bleeding during the immediate posthysterectomy time period. In these instances they became very anxious and concerned about this bleeding. They felt that they were losing control of their bodies and they were afraid that surgery might be necessary to resolve their problem. This complication was successfully resolved by the administration of several blood transfusions. One woman said she was very apprehensive about receiving blood as she was afraid of contracting the Acquired Immune Deficiency Syndrome (AIDS) virus. In contrast, those informants who experienced bladder infections were concerned about their problem but they did not feel threatened by it as they had experienced bladder infections before undergoing the hysterectomy.

Visitors were reportedly disturbed by the changes in the behavior of the women and by the unfamiliar equipment present in the hospital environment. They coped with their anxiety by talking with the informants and also by touching them. Touching behaviors were used most often when the informants experienced severe physical symptoms:

I remember the day of the surgery, as much as I remember. I remember my mom being there, and she kept wiping my brow with a wet cloth 'cause I told her I didn't feel good. I kept saying it really hurt, and she was the most, she was your typical mom. She was there rubbing me and always touching me and making sure I was okay, and I know at one point I looked up to her, and I guess I must have looked really terrible because she looked at me and she just started crying. It was really sad.

As the physical symptoms subsided the informants gradually regained their physical strength and autonomy and required less assistance to carry out daily activities such as bathing and walking. The use of pain killers gradually decreased, reducing the side-effects and enabling the informants to think and relate to their bodies and the outside world in a known, ordinary, and normal fashion.

Observing the Changes

At this point the informants spent time considering the finality of having a hysterectomy. They expressed relief that their previously unacceptable life-style and the hysterectomy were now behind them, but they also experienced a sense of grief. The meaning of their grief did not center on one specific factor such as the absence of the womb, but it comprised many aspects of their lives. The issues of infertility and intimacy with their husbands were aspects that increased the informants' grief and caused a sense of loss and uncertainty about the future. In contrast, the ability to be productive in the workplace and the ability to cope with family and marital relationship demands gave the informants a sense of hope and "balanced" their grief experience.

The informants resolved their grief by exploring the surgery as well as the long-term implications of the hysterectomy. This strategy helped the informants come to terms with the surgical event. The presence or absence of cancer and information about organs left intact or removed were issues examined by all of the women; however, the informants had difficulty obtaining information about how their bodies reacted and how they were handled during the surgery. Although physicians generally did not elaborate on these issues, the informants thought this information was important because it could explain particular physical symptoms. For example, one informant asked her physician why she had pain in her mouth following surgery. He explained that her body had become very tense when the anaesthesia was first introduced and she had unknowingly bitten her tongue.

In addition to explaining particular physical symptoms, knowing how their bodies reacted and how health professionals handled their bodies represented information that reassured the informants. Although their loss of control had been complete, this knowledge confirmed that the health professionals had remained vigilant, respectful of their bodies, and in control of the surgical event:

> It's not so much the part of losing something as it is, you know, not really knowing exactly what they're doing to it, and it's odd. You don't really think about that till it's starting to happen, and then you realize it. You want to know. You just feel odd just turning your body over to somebody. I knew that I had given them permission to do whatever they felt was best for my health, but you expect them to tell you afterward and let you know exactly what happened.

Information about aspects of the surgery helped the informants anticipate the occurrence of particular long-term consequences, for example hormonal instability. Furthermore, the manner in which such information was communicated to them as well as the reactions of others influenced how the informants viewed themselves following the surgery. For example, the informants felt they were less than ordinary women when they thought health professionals and others were indifferent to their situation:

> I said, "How was everything?" And that's when he told me that he had to take everything. He didn't tell me what was really wrong. He didn't tell me what the size was or how everything else was inside, nothing. He just said, "We had to take it all [the uterus and ovaries]." And I don't think that's very fair. I mean, it's my body not his. I was depressed that they had to take it all, but I think I was more upset about the way he talked to me about it. I mean, he's a good doctor, and I'm not really having any problems, you know. It's just that to me it just seemed like I was a number, an assembly line thing, and I don't think doctors should be like that.

As the *Observing the Changes* phase reached completion the informants prepared to return home. Some of their concerns about the future were clarified, although others required a waiting period. For instance, the informants worried about their ability to enjoy sex and this anxiety could not be immediately resolved as they were told to wait up to six weeks before resuming sexual activities.

The informants were given written and/or verbal instructions about activities to avoid in order to ensure a prompt return to a healthy state. Generally the informants did not feel the written information was helpful and the application of some of these instructions was considered unrealistic by many of the informants, especially those with young children and those who had little help in the home. On the other hand, verbal instructions were considered useful because there was opportunity for verbal exchange and clarification. Also, some physicians instructed a few of the informants to listen to or read their bodies and these informants felt this information was useful because their physicians were encouraging the application of a known, ordinary pattern of behavior to promote recovery.

Stage III: Recovering

Adjusting to Changes

After their discharge from the hospital the informants said they began to concentrate on returning to normal. The presence of physical limitations such as abdominal tenderness, constipation, and fatigue needed to be managed and resolved in order for the informants to recover their sense of autonomy and independence. The strategies the informants used to enhance healing involved frequent rest periods, the reestablishment of known bowel and bladder patterns, appropriate nutrition, a gradual increase in activities, and the delegation of tasks to others.

The informants measured healing by observing their body, comparing their body to others, contrasting their present body state to its preoperative state, testing their tolerance to physical activity, and evaluating their body's reactions. When the informants engaged in physical activities they focused on specific areas and functions of their bodies, for example the abdominal area, the incision line, the points of insertion of foreign objects (such as intravenous and intramuscular injection sites), and bowel, bladder, sleep, and appetite patterns.

Over time most of the informants began noticing positive changes in their bodies such as weight stabilization, weight loss, a flattened abdominal area, a fading incision line, bladder control, the absence of presurgical symptoms, an increasing level of energy, and a higher tolerance to stress. The informants said they felt "good" about their bodies and had a greater sense of freedom, especially when changes extended beyond known boundaries of normality:

> I still got my same temper and everything, but something really has to happen to get me in a bad mood. Like before, it didn't take nothing. I just switched from one mood to the other with no reasoning, no nothing behind it, so that plays on your mind, too. You think you're going crazy.

In contrast, some of the informants noted negative changes in their bodies. When complications occurred these women could not reestablish a normal life; instead of freedom they felt restricted by their bodies:

> Everybody was telling me "Six weeks you'll be feeling great." Well, six weeks have come and gone a long time ago, and I'm still not in control of my body, and I think that's part of my anger right now. I'm angry because I'm supposed to be feeling better. This is supposed to be all over with. Now this lump again has got me scared, and I feel like I'm still out of control, and I just don't know when it's going to stop.

When their health continued to improve the informants felt positive about their hysterectomy. A steady improvement confirmed that the decision to undergo surgery had been the right one. In contrast, when complications occurred and when pressures to resume roles were high the informants questioned the decision to have a hysterectomy. In these instances the informants thought the pace of improvement was too slow and they doubted their decision.

Increased pressures to resume roles as well as low access to support resources limited the application of strategies to promote healing for some of the informants in this study. Husbands who did not assist with household tasks and were absent from the home due to work as well as limited assistance from extended family members and friends prevented these informants from implementing and maintaining strategies to heal their bodies.

Women with young children were more limited in their attempts to promote healing than women with older children or without children. Mothers of young children were reluctant to delegate the care of their children to others and they often resumed caregiving as soon as they returned home. The informants said that their children's disrupted sleep patterns, increased irritability, reactions to perceived rejection, and increased demands for touch, attention, and affection were the results of their time in the hospital. These women experienced a conflict between using time-consuming self-care strategies to promote healing and giving time to their children in order to compensate for their absence:

> Like the other day, he hit the corner of the heat register there, and he cut his little head open, and I mean, people say don't lift him up. But I think that was half my problem 'cause I lifted my son way too early, but they don't understand, like, how can you say no to a two year old?

Informants with older children experienced this conflict with less intensity than mothers of small children. Older children had a greater understanding of the situation, more independence, and imposed fewer demands on their mothers during this phase. They demonstrated concern by being more cautious when touching their mothers and they provided support by assisting with tasks in the home.

Although most of the informants said they saw a steady improvement in their health after a few weeks at home, they also experienced times of frustration, boredom, and anxiety. They had control in delegating tasks to others but they had little control over how these tasks were carried out. Family members did not necessarily perform household tasks in the manner desired by the informants and sometimes they justified their actions by criticizing the *way* the informants accomplished tasks around the home. These situations were frustrating and the informants became impatient to resume full management of the family.

Promoting healing involved resuming roles gradually. As a result, the informants had to alter normal patterns of activity during this phase. They had to find new ways to fill the days and manage their boredom. Being bored motivated them to carry out activities that would minimize this feeling and at the same time promote healing. The informants found it difficult to achieve a balance in these areas and others did not always understand the purpose of their activities:

You see, I cleaned the car last night because I wanted to be outside, yet I didn't want to just sit out there. Like the other day, this is really scary, I weeded my deck. . . . There was little weeds growing out of the cracks. I weeded it. My mom phoned me that night. "What were you doing today?" I said, "Weeding the deck." "Have you been smoking something? Were you smoking those weeds?" I said, "No mom." She said, "Why did you weed your deck?" I said, "Because it needed it." My mom really thinks that the doctors took something out here [points to head] when they were down there. It's like, "No mom, it's called finding things to do to keep my sanity," and that's exactly what it is. I know it is because I wouldn't normally weed my deck.

The informants in this study found family roles harder to reclaim than roles in the larger community and workplace. In some instances support resources were limited and the informants had to quickly resume roles within the family. But in other cases assuming normal roles was discouraged by family members as they had difficulty relinquishing activities assumed when the informant was hospitalized. These family members questioned the informants' ability to resume their normal activities, and these particular informants had to justify their readiness verbally or by other means:

I changed my living room around two weeks ago. My husband came home and just about shot me. . . . He said, "Good Christ, it's been that way for years, it can stay that way." But I think it looks much nicer now, there's more room in it.

Community-based roles and roles held in the workplace were resumed with greater ease. The informants said they did not reenter these roles until they had resumed their normal family activities and they said that employers and individuals in the community supported them by encouraging them to carry out activities at their own pace.

Resuming Sexual Activities

The informants experienced anxiety about sexuality during the recovery phase. Because the women had been instructed to wait approximately six weeks before resuming sex they had time to reflect and worry about how they would function sexually. Although all of the informants had been informed about what had been removed from their bodies, most of them had difficulty conceptualizing sexual activities without a uterus. The informants were concerned about what happened to the desire for sex after surgery as well as what happened to the body space previously occupied by the womb.

Those informants who had a close relationship with their physician coped differently with their sexual concerns than those who did not have a close relationship with their physician. Prior to the hysterectomy all of the informants had been told that their sex drive and the pleasure derived from sexual intercourse would remain intact and might even be enhanced as presurgery symptoms would be absent. This information was sufficient to reduce anxiety for the informants who had close relationships with their physicians. In these instances the informants completely trusted their doctor and believed this information was true. In contrast, this information was not sufficient to decrease anxiety for those women who had not established a close relationship with their doctor. In these cases the informants questioned whether their physician told them the truth about their sex life. Furthermore, these women developed a variety of beliefs about resuming sexual activities and about their bodies such as believing that sensations would be different for both the man and the woman as there would be an empty space inside the body, pain was a possibility for the woman as remaining structures might be sutured together, and the sexual drive could be decreased or absent as the uterus might in some way play a role in producing desire. These informants said they wished to know if their assumptions were correct; however, they felt embarrassed about specifically describing them to their physicians. Consequently, these informants experienced a high level of anxiety.

All of the informants resumed sexual activities after a follow-up visit to their physician. The knowledge that healing was progressing as it should and that sexual intercourse could now be safely resumed reassured the husbands because they had been concerned about causing pain or injury to their wives. Although all of the informants still experienced various degrees of anxiety about their sexuality, they were pleased that the opportunity to confront it was finally at

hand. By carefully and gently resuming sexual activities the informants were able to test for the existence of presurgery symptoms
associated with sexual intercourse as well as previously identified
concerns and assumptions.

Most of the informants said their fears and assumptions about
sexual activities were unfounded and they generally had positive
feelings about their sexuality. They experienced pleasure during
sexual activities, but they also perceived some differences in terms
of sensations. Some commented that during penetration it felt tighter
inside. Others said that when penetration occurred they had a tender
area in the lower abdomen, but they added that this particular
sensation decreased over time. One woman reported that she experienced little pleasure during sexual activities and added that she was
just happy that now at least there was no pain. One other informant
in this study expressed negative feelings about her sexuality. This
woman was experiencing complications from her surgery and she
was anxious and concerned about her sexuality and her body. She
said her level of energy and desire for sex were low and she added
that she did not feel sexy because she did not like the appearance
of her body.

The Follow-up Visit to the Physician

During the follow-up visits to physicians information related to the
examination and analysis of tissues removed during the surgical
event were presented and briefly discussed with the informants.
The physicians identified abnormalities such as fibroids, adhesions,
cysts, and venous congestion as probable causal factors of presurgery symptoms. In addition, all of the women were informed that no
cancerous cells had been identified. This knowledge provided the
informants with a final confirmation that the choice for surgery had
been the right decision. One woman reported that her physician did
not identify any abnormalities and said that her uterus had been
normal. In spite of the fact that presurgery symptoms were now
absent she was very disturbed by this information and experienced
doubts about her decision to have a hysterectomy. Causal factors
were not proposed by her physician and she questioned the validity
of her perceptions of the presurgery symptoms.

Coming to Terms with the Hysterectomy

All of the informants in this study attempted to come to terms with their hysterectomy by evaluating their recovery and by seeking evidence that undergoing surgery had been the right decision. The strategies that the informants used to evaluate their recovery included monitoring the healing of their bodies, assessing their energy level after resuming roles and activities, and obtaining the doctor's expert opinion on their progress.

In order to come to terms with their hysterectomy experience the informants attempted to confirm two specific issues directly related to the decision for surgery. The first issue concerned the identification of the cause of the health problem. The informants sought to identify the causal factors of their illness during the follow-up visit with physicians and when causal factors were provided the women were reassured that the decision for surgery had been correct. The second issue that the informants examined was their level of input in the hysterectomy decision-making process. This issue was very important as it enabled the informants to determine if the decision for surgery had or had not been their own. The knowledge that the decision had been their own confirmed their competence in managing their health problem when the recovery was successful and it moderated the effect on their self-esteem when the recovery was unsuccessful. Variations related to the informants' success in coming to terms with their experiences of hysterectomy are presented in Figure 3.8.

Several of the informants had successful recoveries and were satisfied with their decision for surgery (Figure 3.8, Cell *a*). These informants were often surprised by how quickly they recovered from the surgery. They felt they had made the right decision and had dealt with their health problem in a competent manner. In these instances their input in the hysterectomy decision-making process was high. Furthermore, all of these informants were supported during their recovery. Consequently, they were successful in coming to terms with their hysterectomy:

> I zipped right through this one. I was sitting there the other day, and I said, "Geez, it's been over two months boy and back in shape already." That worked out better than I thought it would.

> I think, geez you know, I can never have another one [baby], but for my

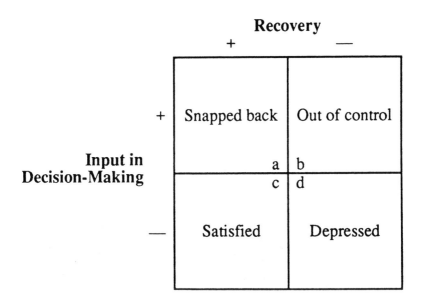

Figure 3.8. Women's Perceptions of the Hysterectomy

health, I'm glad I did it. There's no regrets. I can really honestly say that I'm glad I did it.

I recovered quicker from this than I did from my two C-sections.

Although one woman was satisfied with her decision for surgery, she experienced complications during the recovery (Figure 3.8, Cell *b*). These unforeseen complications impeded her ability to maintain a sense of competence about her situation; in addition maintaining a sense of competence was further hindered by the fact that she had limited support from her husband because he often worked outside the city. She felt out of control and in spite of her extensive involvement in the hysterectomy decision-making process she began to doubt her decision to have the surgery. Because she questioned her competence in dealing with her health problem she also felt devalued as a person and expressed this loss of self-esteem as "not feeling like a woman." Consequently, this informant was unable to come to terms with her surgery:

I feel like maybe I should have thought this through more. I did think it through. I thought I really talked it out with my husband. We decided this would be the best for me, and now. . . . Maybe what I did was wrong.

Other informants were successful in their recovery and they received evidence during the follow-up visit with their physicians that confirmed their decision for surgery had been correct (Figure 3.8, Cell *c*). In addition they were supported during the *Recovering Stage*. These women, however, had very little input in the hysterectomy decision-making process. Consequently, although they felt satisfied that the right decision had been made, they were unable to feel competent about how they had managed their health problem:

I did speak to a lady from another town that had it done, and she said the same thing. She had pretty well the same problem as me, which was comforting to know. I think that was the first person that I'd talked to with the same kind of problem as mine, and she says the same as me, like she never regretted it.

One informant had a successful recovery but was not satisfied with the decision for surgery (Figure 3.8, Cell *d*). In this instance this woman had little input in the hysterectomy decision-making process and she was unable to confirm that the decision for surgery had been the right choice as her physician could not identify the causal factors of her illness. Furthermore, she was not supported during her recovery. Like the informant who experienced complications during her recovery from the hysterectomy (Figure 3.8, Cell *b*), this informant was unable to feel competent about how she had managed her health problem and she continued to review the decision to have a hysterectomy. Although her physical recovery was successful, she did not perceive it as such and she was depressed about her situation because she felt she had not appropriately assessed and dealt with her symptoms. Consequently, she felt devalued as a person and could not come to terms with her surgery:

I feel so sad. I feel so empty inside, you know. . . . Towards my younger baby, I feel like I have to stick with her all the time. It's just an unbelievable feeling. I never felt that way before.

A successful recovery and the confirmation that the decision to have a hysterectomy had been correct were events that signified that life was back to normal for the women in this study. Those who could not confirm that their decision to have a hysterectomy was correct, however, and those who experienced an unsuccessful recovery were unable to come to terms with their surgery and did not feel their lives were back to normal.

Note

1. This investigation involved a total of 10 women who had undergone a hysterectomy within the previous month, and they were selected from a large teaching hospital. The informants were interviewed at one and three months posthysterectomy. The informants ranged in age from 24 to 39 years and all but one were married. All of the women with the exception of one had children. A total of 18 interviews, lasting from 45 to 90 minutes, were conducted with these informants.

4

Becoming Ordinary:
Leaving the Psychiatric Hospital

BEVERLEY LORENCZ

A significant problem in qualitative research is trying to understand the patient's perspective when the patient is unable to speak or to express him- or herself. If the patient is unable to speak (as in the case of preverbal infants or aphasic adults) the researcher is forced to use observational techniques such as participant-observation or ethology. Both of these techniques involve a certain amount of researcher inference when the research question pertains to patient feelings. If the patient is able to speak but is confused, glimpses of the patient's reality may be obtained through interviews if the researcher has extraordinary skill and patience, especially when the researcher is competing with the multiple voices and realities with which the delusional patient must contend. The value of this latter approach is evident in this chapter.

Lorencz's thesis committee members recognized the problems associated with using a verbal technique with patients who may not be able to express themselves, and she was strongly recommended not to undertake her study on the experiences of adults with schizophrenia who are about to be discharged. Despite this recommendation she continued with this onerous study to the amazement and awe of her thesis committee members. One of the most crucial qualities of an excellent researcher (along with creativity, sensitivity, and wisdom) is perseverance. Perseverance is the most essential quality of a researcher in that it

AUTHOR'S NOTE: Derived from: Lorencz, B. J. (1988). *Perceptions of adult chronic schizophrenics during planned discharge.* Unpublished master's thesis, University of Alberta, Edmonton, Alberta, Canada.

This research was supported in part by grants from the Alberta Association of Registered Nurses and the Alberta Foundation for Nursing Research.

assures completion of a difficult project and enables the researcher to prove that certain data are obtainable despite overwhelming odds. When conducting the interviews for this study Lorencz often waited for more than a minute for responses to her questions. When these responses came they often were responses to another voice—an internal voice—and as a result the interview often seemed nonsensical, slow, and convoluted. Throughout data collection these apparently irrelevant glimpses into the experiences of these patients were interpreted not as nonsensical delusions, but as the informant's own reality. As a result a creative and powerful grounded theory emerged from this study.

Schizophrenia has been referred to as the "cancer of psychiatry" (Green, 1984). Only 50% of those diagnosed with schizophrenia are expected to achieve either a complete or good recovery (Bland, 1984). Whereas at one time schizophrenics were institutionalized on a long-term basis, they are now encouraged to live in the community. Research has revealed, however, that the majority of schizophrenics require repeated hospitalizations (Bland, Parker, & Orn, 1976, 1978; Cottman & Mezey, 1976). The repeated admissions of schizophrenics is known as "the revolving door syndrome."

The past decade has witnessed the development of several community programs for schizophrenics; however, the persistently high admission rates attest to the failure of these programs. Although much research has been published about discharged schizophrenics the researchers have examined the problem from the perspective of the care provider. In order to plan and implement effective community-based treatment an understanding of the schizophrenics' experiences must be gained. Schizophrenics in the community are "free-agents" and the programs planned must meet their needs and address their concerns, not just the concerns of health professionals. Therefore, a study was conducted to examine the perceptions of predischarge chronic schizophrenics who have experienced at least two years of illness.[1]

Preadmission Experiences: Being a Failure

Individuals do not become psychiatric inpatients solely due to the existence of mental hospitals. Although psychiatric admissions may coincide with the application of the label *mentally ill,* numerous factors interact before culminating in these admissions. One factor is the patient's prehospitalization functioning. The informants in this study consistently characterized their preadmission functioning as inadequate. Their perceptions of their failure to function in the community combined with the assigned meaning of their admission to the hospital produced the context for the occurrence of the process of *becoming ordinary.* This chapter begins with a review of the informants' preadmission experiences and the meanings they assigned to their hospital admissions.

The informants in this study divided their preadmission experiences into two periods of time: the extended past and the preadmission past. The pivotal point which demarcates these periods of time from each other is the participants' first contact with mental health care (please note that "I" stands for Informant and "R" stands for Researcher):

I: Then I had a lot of freedom. And then all of the sudden, wham, I'm stuck up in a hospital, and I was changed. I was—I didn't—I didn't give a damn for awhile, eh? And then, and then, it got harder, even harder. And then the doctors got at me, and that's where I'm at. The doctors are talking about me, eh? What they think I am, and what they think, feel I want, and what I—what I do, and what I think, and stuff like that.

R: What ways is the atmosphere "not peaceful"?

I: I don't know. Until I went home, I use to hang around with some really good friends, and I found that really relaxing and peaceful. And then I went home and, ah, I ran into this mental health stuff. And I can't say I've had a peaceful moment since.

R: You haven't had a peaceful moment since you've been involved with mental health people?

I: That's right.

R: What's been happening?

I: Uh, I get deeper and deeper into quicksand, I guess.

R: You feel you're deeper in quicksand?

I: Yeah, there's no way out.

R: I don't understand. There's no way out of . . .

I: Out of mental health.

The themes underlying the two periods of time that constitute the past are different. The extended past is best characterized as "the good old days." Conversely, the participants' preadmission past is an extended period of *not making it* in the community culminating in the informants' present admission. The preadmission past, which includes previous hospitalizations, ranges from approximately three to fifteen years, and the preadmission past is contingent upon the past psychiatric history of the informant.

The Extended Past

Events recalled from the extended past are characteristically experiences that illustrate successful management in the community. The informants primarily recalled two types of experiences: previous interpersonal relationships and occupational experiences:

> Uh huh, someone to come home to. When I worked on the rigs, I was living common-law. I'd come home after work, there'd be a bacon and tomato sandwich there and a beer. The little boy, he'd be jumping and rolling around, giggling, and squealing, and cooing. [pause] And, ah, it made me feel like a man. [pause] Made me feel real good. Like you'd come home after sweating and working your muscles real hard, getting screamed at by some ratty driller.

> I had a heck of a time on the first couple of rigs I was working on. Finally, I hit one I liked. That was, ah, a step up sub. I got offered a drilling job on one of them, at one time. That's how come I like them.

Although recalled events might have occurred in the distant past, the informants often spoke about them as though they had occurred recently. For example, one informant's interviews were dominated by his recollections of his experiences as a laborer. He frequently spoke as if these events had occurred in the recent past. Clarification revealed that these events had occurred more than ten years prior to the interview:

I: Actually, it was tough with that rig. But then I had my cement forms in mind. I had worked for, eh, eighteen months on a drilling rig straight. Seven hours, no, well, it would be seven days a week for eighteen months. And I just wanted to get away.

R: You'd get pretty tired?

I: Yeah, I was pretty sick of drilling rigs.
R: Was that two years ago when you quit?
I: No, that was, ah, back when I was about twenty-three years old.

Two further points can be made about the data gained from the informants in this study. First, the informants did not reminisce about childhood days with their families. They predominantly recalled experiences away from home, or, if still living at home, experiences with their school peers. Second, the informant with the longest history of previous psychiatric care made the fewest references to the extended past. In comparison to the more recent histories of the other informants (three to four years), this informant had a fifteen year history of psychiatric care and his references to the extended past were limited to relating illicit drug experiences shared with his peers:

> We had the sense not to smoke drugs, hash or marijuana, after we were on acid because we're an elite. We were, we were in [a] generation that was lost in space. We, we had things to do, and we did them.

The Preadmission Past

The preadmission past is best characterized as a long period of *not making it* in the community accompanied by feelings of discouragement, loneliness, and a sense of being overwhelmed. Some of the informants initiated compensatory behaviors to alleviate these feelings; however, these behaviors were often dysfunctional because the outcome tended to deepen their feelings of alienation and thereby compounded their sense of isolation from the greater community.

Not Making It

The informants defined *not making it* as inadequate functioning in the community: "Ah, I didn't think I'd get mentally thick—sick. I thought I'd be able to function." The yardstick generally used to measure their ability to function in the community was social norms, which the informants unquestioningly accepted as appropriate standards for self-evaluation:

I: Kind of instead of going against the grains of society, I'll go along with it.

R: Do you consider yourself going, as in the past, as going against the grains?

I: Yeah, with a name like ____, I sure do.

R: What are the grains of society, going with the grains of society? What does that mean?

I: Um, laughter, I suppose, and money, [pause] comfortably involved with endeavors.

A second informant said he had deviated from "the norm, from the righteous side of society":

R: We were talking about before you went into ____, you were doing a lot of drugs and alcohol and you flipped out. Can you kind of describe what's flipped out. What happens when you flip out?

I: Being out of the norm from the righteous side of society. [pause] When you do that, you become persecuted by yourself and the people around you.

Self-comparisons were occasionally made with others in the community whom the informants felt had achieved the social norms for functioning:

You can always say that you're gonna make, make something out something, but it doesn't always work. That's, that's the bugger. It's different, it's strange 'cause when—my brothers and sisters are all super people. Like not super people, but they all can make something work for them and I can't. I don't know. I don't know why. It's amazing. I've been trying.

Community members (including peers) whom the informants felt did not emulate these norms were rejected as yardsticks for comparison. One informant described his previous peer group in the community as "the dregs of society" because the group members abused drugs and alcohol. Discharged psychiatric patients living in the community were also rejected as standards for comparison:

You see, I spent some time in another group home. . . . It's not nice at all because you realize that people that are there . . . are there because of the same reason you're there.

The informants based their evaluation of not making it in the community on their retrospective appraisal of their personal well-being while residing in the community. They recalled both their level of functioning and the accompanying mental well-being.

Self-Evaluation of Community Functioning

All of the informants in this study characterized their preadmission functioning in the community as inadequate. They identified two areas of inadequate functioning: employment and intimate interpersonal relationships. Only one informant expressed satisfaction with the quality of his preadmission peer relationships. The majority of informants expressed feelings of loneliness and this lack of a sense of fellowship in the community resulted from either the absence of companionship or the presence of nonsupportive peers in the community:

R: And you find it not such a good idea being alone?
I: Nah, I miss half of the world. Sleep through half and miss another half . . . the whole world goes by.
I: My friends generally persecute me. They thought I was a joke.
R: They thought you were a joke?
I: Uh huh, they'd play my emotions that way, find a weak spot and tease me about it. It's just a subtle way of giving me strength. . . . By joking about somebody's inadequacies, you give them strength. Although you may frustrate them and put them down, but, eventually, you gain strength from the situation.

Unfortunately, the presence of peers in the community cannot be equated with the availability of emotional support. Although this informant felt his peers were helping him by rejecting his behavior, he did not identify this peer group as supportive. He complained of feeling "loneliness to the max" when he attempted to quit smoking marijuana. He also stated that being mentally ill is being frustrated: "You can't reveal your emotions properly—somebody to care about or somebody that will listen."

Employment was the second area of inadequate community functioning identified by the informants in this study. The informants in this study were young adult males in their twenties and thirties, and from their perspective, the fundamental aspect of *not making it* in the community was their failure to be self-supporting. Only one informant had been employed during the previous two years. He described his job in a convenience store as "boring" and "unfulfilling." Due to termination from his place of employment, this informant had been receiving unemployment insurance for the past year.

The informants were ambivalent about accepting supplementary sources of financial support. Although they recognized their need for this assistance, they thought social assistance was unearned income:

R: It sounds like you don't particularly like being on it [pension].
I: In some ways, it's necessary; in some ways, it's a hand out.
R: Can you tell me more about that?
I: Well, you don't ever have to worry about being fired. So the stress there is gone, so it's beneficial that way. Ah, getting something for nothing has always disturbed me, so it's negative in that way. That's my only beef about being on it.

Self-Evaluation of Mental Well-Being

The predominate emotional state recalled by the informants is congruous with their perceived functioning in the community. All the informants referred to feeling overwhelmed while residing in the community. Some of them explicitly identified stress as the underlying basis for these feelings:

I never missed a day of work, you know. And things were really piling up on me, you know, a lot of stress and stuff like that. My hair was just falling out. You should have seen that. I could go like this [running fingers through his hair]. I could go like this with my [showed researcher hand with hair between the fingers] like that, and have about ten hairs.

Other informants implicated stress in their descriptions of being overwhelmed. These informants recalled feeling "bogged down," being in a "real panic," "everything was moving kind of fast anyway, just not enough time," and "the whole world was upside down there for a little while."

The level of stress experienced by the informants was not temporarily related to their admissions; instead, they described this stress as chronic and encompassing the entire preadmission period. For example, although the preadmission past included previous psychiatric hospitalizations, the informants did not describe a transient period of reduced stress following these discharges:

R: How about the other times when you left, how did you feel then?
I: I felt good. I felt good that I was leaving, but I wasn't as certain as I am now, you know. Like I thought, I didn't think I'd come back, but you know, but, but I still had the problems. I was just on a fake medication, you know. They had me on the wrong meds, and, um, it was just a phony reality. Really, because I was walking around in a daze all day. That's 'cause I was on pretty heavy medication, you know.

A second informant spoke of his anticipated success following treatment:

I took Assertiveness Training and I thought, "Ah, ah, I got it made, I can set myself in any direction I want" and then, it's people that get to me, eh. It's the people, it's not the—maybe it is the surroundings. I dunno.

Being Overwhelmed

The informants identified factors which intensified or precipitated feelings of being overwhelmed in the community. These factors are categorized into two main groups: the informants' behaviors and environmental influences. Environmental influences are further subdivided into nonintrusive and intrusive influences.

Environmental Influences

Environmental influences are those influences that the informants identified as having an external origin. Intrusive influences encompassed intrusions into the informants' cognitive sphere by either known or unknown others. One informant described intrusive experiences as "things that aren't there, but pop in there, out of thin air." Nonintrusive influences were events/conditions occurring in the informants' objective environment.

Intrusive Influences

Mental health professionals consider intrusive influences an intra-psychic phenomenon, a cardinal sign of psychosis; however, the informants in this study who experienced this phenomenon did not accept this premise:

> And, ah, I was laying on my bed and I was—I felt like I was dying. It was this patient next to me cursing me to death. And I was resentful for what he said. And, ah, I felt like my spirit was leaving my body.

This experience occurred prior to this informant's transfer from a community hospital. Another informant also experienced mental intrusion by a known other. He initially expressed disbelief at what was happening:

> Okay, okay, just listen to me, okay. That's all I ask. And, um, one day, I was, I was sitting in bed and I was thinking about ____, you know. And I, I felt really bad about it, and everything like that. And I just started crying, eh? And, um, all of sudden, all of sudden, all my thoughts were being displayed, you know. I could hear my thoughts being said. And then I asked them, I asked them through my mind. I said "How, how, how do, [are] you doing this?" and they told me "ESP." And I said "That's bullshit, I don't believe in ESP." And they said, "Some people have this special gift," you know, and it was really amazing.

Although health care professionals categorize such experiences as intrapsychic, the informants in this study believed they were externally generated. Furthermore, they continued to conceive of these experiences as interpersonal problems throughout their hospitalization. The following quote illustrates how the informants envisaged them as relationship problems rather than indicators of psychological problems:

R: So when you'd go out, what would happen?
I: I'd drink a little bit too much [laugh] and get really plastered and forget to take my meds, and then I'd get sick again and terrible.

R: What sort of things happened when you got sick again?
I: Um . . . I was just hearing really bad voices and, um, telling me really
     strange things, bizarre things. And I'd believe them, and I'd get sick, you
     know. They'd make me really sick.

For this informant the presence of the voices was not indicative of illness; rather, illness resulted from his relationship with the voices, that is, he believed them.

The informants' feelings of being overwhelmed were directly and indirectly magnified by intrusive experiences. The informants who experienced these phenomena described direct changes in their mental well-being, which they attributed to the effect of these experiences. One informant said he felt "stifled" during these intrusive experiences and another informant described himself as "mentally restricted":

Um, I was restricted because I felt that there was people reading my thoughts and, um, you know, and knew what I was doing, and everything like that, you know. And that use to bother me a lot. So I couldn't really function the way I want to function, eh.

This informant also described experiencing an extended period of "total depression" while residing in the community.

All of the informants considered these intrusions a restrictive burden and as a result of these intrusions the informants had fewer personal resources available for dealing with their nonintrusive surroundings as their personal resources were used to manage the intrusive experiences. The informants' methods for managing intrusive experiences will be described later in this chapter.

Nonintrusive Influences

Nonintrusive influences are the second type of environmental factors identified by the informants in this study. Nonintrusive influences are burdensome events/conditions occurring within the informants' objective environment. The two major categories of nonintrusive influences affecting the informants' sense of mental well-being (which were examined earlier in this chapter) were the lack of paid employment and the lack of supportive interpersonal relationships in the community. Each of these influences contributed to the informants' sense of declining mental well-being in several ways.

The informants described feelings of inadequacy and failure arising from their inability to obtain long-term employment. Two of the informants attributed their failure to obtain paid employment to the lack of understanding employers in the community: "Like, I'm not lazy, and I like to work, but I just, I can't, I can't connect on a good job or [a] patient employer." As well, losing a job adversely affected the informants' confidence in their abilities to function in the community.

> I use to work in a glass factory in ____. . . . The guy knew damn well that I was sick, eh, and so he gave me the boot. The same with, um, the same with the—it sort of makes me wonder about myself. Just what—where I am, and what kind of functions I do have, you know.

The informants experienced several stressful incidents due to their lack of supportive relationships in the community. These incidents involved the rejection of the informants' behavior by significant others, for example rejection by members of community institutions (such as churches), requests by family members to seek alternative living arrangements, and, finally, rejection by peers.

The informants did not feel supported by their community. Half of the informants related incidents of perceived rejection by other community members: "Sometimes, you see, I get the strangest looks. . . . I'm not gonna worry about it. I's too bad for them." Another informant described himself as a "modern day leper":

> As soon as someone finds out you've got a disease of the mind, they right away start treating you as a second class citizen. As if they're superior 'cause they're somewhat more normal than you are.

The majority of the informants identified specific aspects or events in their social environment which contributed significantly to their feelings of being overwhelmed, for example rejection by significant others. There was one exception to this: The participant with the longest history of previous psychiatric care indiscriminately described the social community outside the hospital as threatening and punitive. This informant believed that the community was composed of powerful, malevolent others:

If I, if I try to do something, there's always someone out there, that, that's there to outsmart me, you know. So, I gotta be careful. I gotta—I can't just give up, right?

Behavioral Influences

The informants said the misuse of drugs and alcohol intensified or precipitated feelings of being overwhelmed in the community. All of the informants described drug and alcohol related experiences. Although the majority of the informants described continuous use of these substances throughout the preadmission period, one inform-ant said his use of alcohol was limited to the extended past. Although environmental influences such as peer group pressure were present for some informants, all of them felt they voluntarily used these substances.

The informants accounted for their use of drugs and alcohol in two ways. First, for some of the informants the use of drugs and alcohol was an expected and acceptable peer group behavior.

> In the group I was dealing with it was socially acceptable, and it made me feel good, sometimes paranoid. It would strengthen the ties between me and my friends, so I became to be dependent on them, the dope and the company. It was a socializing skill.

Second, the informant described the use of drugs and alcohol as an accessible method for reducing feelings of insecurity as well as for helping them persevere in the community. For the informants the use of these substances was a means for gaining temporary respite from life in the community:

> I like smoking hash, you know. It keeps me, it keeps me going. I don't get burnt out and stuff like that. . . . But I like smoking dope, and it's a great antidepressant.

> It's just something to get me away from where I am.

Another informant said the use of drugs and alcohol alleviated his feelings of insecurity and enhanced his sense of fellowship with his peers:

> R: When you say it helped you feel good, in what sort of ways?

I: I was able to relax, it took away the frustration.
R: Frustration from . . .
I: Self-insecurities.
I: I felt more at one with people in the room. I could carry out a conversation better.

When the intended effect was not achieved the use of drugs and alcohol was detrimental to the informants; however, any adverse effects were not attributed to the use of these substances but to their misuse:

I was drinking too much. I'd drink every day. I was, I was nearly an alcoholic by the time I got out of that place.

I just take, I just, I overindulge. I just do too much of—I go to the bar, I drink myself crazy.

This overuse of drugs and alcohol adversely affected the respondents' mental well-being:

R: It helped you relax?
I: Right. Actually, it added stress in certain cases too. People get paranoid when they use a lot of dope.
R: Uh huh, what does it mean to "get paranoid"?
I: Oh, cold, clammy physically, and your thoughts racing mentally.

The informants also reported isolated, indirect effects of substance overuse. For example, one informant said he would forget to take his prescribed medication when inebriated and as a result of failing to comply with his drug therapy he would hear "really bad voices." Only one informant reported experiencing negative feelings associated with the use of illegal substances: "Guilt because you're breaking the law. Guilt because you're dependent upon a substance."

Unfortunately, no influences that helped the informants adjust to the community were discussed during the interviews and the informants only identified those factors that precipitated or intensified their feelings of being overwhelmed while residing in the community. For the informants in this study the preadmission period was an extended period of *not making it* in the community.

Also, the informants identified few volitional behaviors that contributed to their perception of *not making it*, and behaviors which others may identify as detrimental to community living (such as violence against others) are excluded because they were not labeled as such by the respondents.

Finally, it was noted earlier that the preadmission period ranged from three to fifteen years and this period was contingent on the informant's history of previous psychiatric care. The identified influences also fit into this extended time period. For example, one informant said he believed that being asked to seek alternative living arrangements precipitated his feelings of being overwhelmed; however, this incident had occurred at least three years prior to his present admission. Personal rejection by a significant other was identified by another informant as a major contributing factor to his sense of social isolation in the community. This rejection had also occurred at least two years prior to his present admission.

Admission to the Hospital

The meaning the informants assigned to their admission to the hospital had behavioral and social implications and involved the integration of three facets of admission to psychiatric hospitals: the level of preadmission functioning, the perceived initiator of admission, and the informant's conception of mental hospitals *per se*. For the informants, being admitted to the hospital meant they were functioning poorly in the community and that their behavior was unacceptable to the greater community.

A factor influencing the meaning assigned to admission was the informants' assessment of their preadmission functioning. The informants described themselves as *not making it* in the community during this period of time. The informants said that during the preadmission period they felt overwhelmed and frustrated. The preadmission period ended with the informant's admission to the hospital.

A second influencing factor was the informants' perception of who initiated their admission. A striking feature apparent in the data was the fact that the informants did not believe their admission was the result of their own actions. This phenomenon was apparent regardless of the informant's admission status: voluntary (i.e., signed self in for treatment) or involuntary (i.e., admission certificates):

And then I got *called back.*

This was why I got *sent here.*

I got *committed.*

He just sent me straight up here. [referring to family physician]

I got taken out the room, the police came, off duty, and, ah, you see there was no evidence. And the next thing I was told [was] "You're beyond our rules, *we're shipping you* to _____." And the next thing I knew, I was in an ambulance and up here.

These quotes are from the informants who were certified at the time of admission. Only one informant in this study voluntarily admitted himself to the hospital. He also described his admission as initiated by others, in this case his father: "*He, he took me* out for a drive away from the home, and *he said to get back* to the place."

The informants' tendency to feel that their admission was initiated by others was present regardless of the events precipitating the admission:

My doctor was sick and tired of me ODing. . . . He was fed up with me, man. He just wasn't gonna take no more of my shit. *He just sent me* straight up here. He called as soon as he found out. He called straight up here. He was very firm with me, you know.

Although this informant had attempted suicide, he still attributed his admission to the actions of his physician. Another informant was admitted following a violent attack on another patient in a city hospital. This informant also did not attribute his admission to his violent behavior; instead, he attributed it to the intervention of others.

Related to this phenomenon was the informants' failure to identify significant events that resulted in the deterioration of their feelings of well-being immediately prior to admission. Although two informants described events that precipitated their admission, they did not describe any deterioration in their sense of well-being prior to these incidents. Both informants described having problems functioning in the community prior to these incidents. For example, the informant whose suicide attempt precipitated his admission described

experiencing an extended period of depression while he was living
in the community:

> It's a terrible feeling living in depression, you know. It really is, um, I've,
> I've lived with it for years, you know. Like months on end I was living in
> total depression, you know.

A third factor influencing the meaning assigned to admission to
the hospital was the informants' perceptions of psychiatric hospitals *per se.* The informants' impressions of psychiatric hospitals
varied and depended on their previous psychiatric treatment. Informants undergoing their first admission to a provincial psychiatric
treatment center became afraid when first informed of their impending admission:

> I: I didn't like it, you know. I, I wondered, "Oh, no, they're sending me to
>   _____, a crazy place," you know. Like you hear so many things about
>   _____, and they're such negative things.
> R: What sort of things did you hear?
> I: Um, just, just like this is a really terrible place to come to and a lot of
>   bad memories from the people that come here, usually come back and
>   stuff like that. Just a lot of negative things, you know.

A second respondent said that coming into the hospital "scared the
hell out of [him]":

> I'd heard all kinds of stories about _____. I was expecting thumb screws
> and stuff like that. . . . Quite scared. I didn't know what to expect. I was
> expecting ECT [electroconvulsive therapy] treatment and large needles
> and lobotomies and stuff like that.

The informants with histories of previous admissions did not
experience this fear. They tended to regard psychiatric care centers
as institutions for people who fail to *make it* in the community. One
informant described the hospital as "just a warehouse to start over,
I guess." A second respondent said he was admitted to hospital
because he "burns out" in the community: "Somehow I can't function
and I can't perform, sort of thing." He also said "it's not too bad"
being admitted to the hospital.

It was indicated earlier that the meaning informants assigned to their admissions has behavioral and social components. Behaviorally, the informants' admissions objectively substantiated their perceptions of themselves as failures:

> I seen my folks, and I broke down in front of my father. I started crying, and he, he took me out for a drive away from the home. And, um, he said to get back to the place. And I said . . . "What about my position in life?" Eh? "Why aren't I such a big success like everyone else?"

Another informant said, "I'm not too proud of the place or myself being in here, I suppose. Just not interested. . . . [It is] just about the bottom."

Socially, the informants in this study felt admission to the hospital symbolized condemnation of their behavior by the greater community: "I thought I was being condemned [by] the government and I would never get out. . . . At least, that's what I thought at the time." Other informants also made reference to feeling that they were being punished by others for their behavior in the community:

> Like I didn't do anything to make it in here. . . . I didn't take anybody's life. I didn't murder anyone. I didn't steal anything. Well, I might of stole a pack of smokes or something from the corner drug store, but nothing.

Only one informant openly expressed resentment toward those he thought were responsible for his admission. He said he "was set up," and he maintained that others in the community display the same behavior that he felt contributed to his admission:

> I get into a fist fight every five or six years, it seems like, or an act of violence of some sort. [pause] And there's other people that I know on the outside that get into fist fights almost daily or bi-daily, and they never get put away.

Consequently, the informants felt that admission to a psychiatric care center represented official redress to their inability to function in the community.

The respondents' preadmission experiences combined with the meaning assigned to hospital admission resulted in the informants entering into a *becoming ordinary* process. This process occurred when the respondents saw themselves as failures in comparison to others or to accepted social norms. All of the respondents emphasized behavioral inadequacies and not psychological difficulties when discussing their preadmission past.

The informants in this study emphasized functional normalcy, not psychological wellness; consequently, *"becoming ordinary"* was used to designate this process in preference to *"becoming normal."* To some normality may imply judgment of the psychological well-being of the informant, but *"becoming ordinary"* does not imply psychological well-being.

Readiness to Return to the Community: "Anticipating Mastery"

The primary criterion for selecting informants for this study was that the informants in cooperation with their treatment team were seeking community placement. Although the informants were selected in accordance with this criterion, it is apparent from the data that the informants' expressed desire to leave the hospital may not have represented their own assessment of their readiness to return to the community. It is also apparent from the data that the meaning the informants assigned to their return to the community was different from the meaning they assigned to the act of being discharged.

All of the informants in this study wanted to leave the hospital. One informant, however, was uncertain about his readiness to reside in the community (see Figure 4.1). In contrast, the other informants anticipated making a successful transition to community living. Although they did not refer to their anticipated future adjustment solely in terms of their ability to manage community demands, these informants were *anticipating mastery* of their posthospital communities. The informants who were *anticipating mastery* were anticipating personal excellence in their pursuit of *ordinary* goals. These informants expected to meet the community's demands and become independent and self-sufficient. For the informants in this study, *anticipating mastery* meant that they could attain their personal goals by meeting the demands of their community.

Desire	Anticipated Functioning	Readiness
#1: I wanted to get the hell out of this hospital that's what I want.	If I was, if I was, ah, to go out in the world, I'd never make it. I just can't, I just can't put it together. I just can't put enough of myself together.	Absent
#2: Ah, I just don't like spending my time in here.	I'm looking — I'm kind of exited about finding a job and earning some money to put in the bank.	Present
#3: I don't, I don't like being here, you know. I'd jump at the chance to get out of here.	Um, I see myself working, and I see myself progressing. I see myself as being simgle and loving every minute of it.	Present
#4: [It's been] long enough. Half a year, half a year to me anyway. That's as much as I want to spend in this place.	In a month from now, I should be on AICSH [pension], working part time, attending programs, getting back into society on an even basis, or a controlled basis rather.	**Present**

Figure 4.1. Comparison of Informant's Desire for Discharge and Anticipated Community Functioning

Indicators of "Anticipating Mastery"

The informants expressed *anticipating mastery* of posthospital communities in three ways: by anticipating a successful transition to community living, by planning concrete strategies for attaining goals in the community, and by expressing positive self-regard.

Anticipating Successful Transition to Community Living

The informants who were *anticipating mastery* felt returning to the community was an opportunity to "start over." In spite of their preadmission failures these informants anticipated positive postdischarge experiences. For the informants in this study discharge did not precede the resumption of life in the community; instead, discharge was seen as the start to a "new life":

It's gonna be a new experience. I'm looking forward to it, and it's gonna be wonderful.

It's a new beginning in the sense that, um, I'm starting my life over. I'm, I'm moving out of the house, and, you know, I'm gonna be going to school and all those things.

Just a new beginning for me anyway. . . . Oh, just starting to hoard things for the future again. Maybe buy a new car or whatever.

These informants also anticipated a successful transition to community living:

It'll be a lot of hard work too, you know. Like, it'll definitely, you know, be its pros and cons, but I'm sure that I'll be able to adjust and fit in right.

I feel most comfortable out in the community right now. After living in a place like that [hospital], I think I'm more than prepared to survive in the community.

I found it hard to make a living before, but now life seems a lot simpler.

These informants also stated they were ready for discharge. One informant said, "I'm just ready to go. I can't put it into words. . . . You know when you're ready to, and I'm ready to go." Another informant reported being "ready and able to deal with myself and society."

Only one of the informants was unequivocal regarding future inpatient treatment. This informant said his problems were resolved and "this time I won't be coming back. Like this is the last time I'll be here. I know that for a fact." The other two informants were uncertain about their need for future hospitalization. This uncertainty was associated with their belief that they might experience a decline in their present state of personal well-being. "I'll never have to come back to a place like this again. If I ever got sick, I hope I don't have to come back to this place."

The fourth informant in this study did not feel his impending return to the community indicated "starting a new life." This informant believed his return to the community was a continuation of his preadmission "struggle to make it":

It's the people that get to me, eh? It's the people, it's not the—maybe it's the surroundings. I dunno. Something's gotta hook on my line or something. Because always when I'm there . . . if I try to do something, there's always someone out there . . . that's there to outsmart me, you know. So I gotta be careful. I gotta. I can't just give up.

This informant did not anticipate a successful transition to community living; instead, he was uncertain about his readiness to reside in the community:

Probably end up back here in another half year. Will be some tiny . . . incident at the group home. Either that or 'cause I can't find work. Somehow . . . I can't function, and I can't perform sort of thing.

This informant was also uncertain about his need for future admissions. His uncertainty, however, was associated with a lack of self-confidence about his ability to manage in the community.

The informants' ideas concerning their anticipated community environments did not account for the variance in *anticipating mastery* of these environments.

Anticipated Community Environment

The informants in this study anticipated two types of community environments: nonthreatening, hospitable environments and threatening, malevolent environments. Two informants anticipated a nonthreatening, hospital community environment, and two informants anticipated a threatening, malevolent community environment.

A Nonthreatening, Hospitable Environment

Two informants believed their discharge communities would offer both employment opportunities and emotional support from family members and friends. Although only one of these informants felt this environment would be charitable, neither of the informants thought the environment would be punitive or restrictive:

I got a job waiting for me in ____. I got buckets of money waiting for me in, ah, ____, which is a nice town. I'm closer to the phone. . . . I'm never broke either. I can always phone up service rigs and go to work for them. Um . . . they make about the same. Like, ah, you can work about maybe ten days for a service rig and make a month's pay.

It just goes . . . to say, you know, all you have to do is hold out your hand, you know. If you're in need, that's all you have to do is hold out your hand, and it's given to you. It's a great song, you know. This is a great country. . . . It's a great country, you know. Everything is set up for me, you know. There's, you know, I don't have to be a genius to, you know, survive and nothing like that.

A Threatening, Malevolent Environment

Two informants thought their anticipated community would be threatening and malevolent. They described this environment as containing anonymous, punitive others. One of these informants described the world as "painful" and anticipated requiring daily deprogramming "from all the nasty people" in the community:

I suppose that's the hardest thing that happens to a person during the day, out in society is slander and common assault. . . . [Common assault] is double talking a person when he's having another conversation, [two conversations going on at once] one malicious and one benign.

Somebody that's—what's the word I'm looking for—is, ah, up to date on my problems. Is able to counsel me at the daybreak and the day end. [pause] That's about it. Somebody to deprogram me at the end of the day. . . . Well, everyday somebody gives you certain information, derogatory or positive or whatever. And you just gotta sort the good from the bad and have a good night.

Although this informant said supportive friends were present in his community, he also spoke of being "damned" by the "righteous people. The ones that feel too self-righteous. There's a difference between righteous and self-righteous."

The second informant who anticipated a threatening, malevolent community environment did not identify any sources of emotional support within his discharge community. He felt the world was oppressive and immoral:

You know, like . . . if the world doesn't settle down, like there will be bugs and everything else. People will be putting bugs in people's brains. And it's all a Chinese factor, right? Like the Chinese are out to kill, eh? I don't know why, but they're out to frighten the world, its population and to seduction. It's . . . very terminal. It's . . . you have to be careful or you can get caught in that. Who knows. . . . It's very sin. . . . It's a . . . big sin. It's a large sin, and I don't like it—being part of it. . . . I mean there's . . . a lot of young in the world . . . that are really strong. And, um, and, ah, their power tripping ways take them wherever they wanna go. They power trip at the face of the person.

The first indicator of *anticipating mastery* was anticipating a successful transition to community living. The informants who thought they were ready to return to the community characterized their return as starting over. In contrast, the one informant who did not believe he was ready to return to the community did not see entry into the community as an opportunity to reestablish himself in the community. In fact he did not think his forthcoming discharge would have much impact on his present life course.

Planning Concrete Strategies for Attaining Goals in the Community

The second indicator of *anticipating mastery* was planning concrete strategies for attaining personal goals in the community. Although one informant defined his impending return to the community differently, his long-term aspirations were similar to those expressed by the other informants.

Aspirations

All of the informants wanted to achieve a sense of personal achievement in the community. Prior to their admissions they occupied marginal, dependent community roles. At predischarge they expressed a desire to become productive, self-supporting community members:

It's my turn . . . to give back to society. . . . I've taken so much, why not return it? I've lived my life in sin, and I'm not afraid to admit it. It's about time I did something good for the world.

I'll do it. I have lots of time yet, but, you know, but I wanna start producing and making some constructive progressions in life.

I wanna work. I wanna get back. I wanna work in the work force. I wanna work for a living, earn a living.

The majority of the informants preferred manual labor employment; only one informant aspired to become a professional. This informant, however, planned to finance his education by working in restaurants. The places of employment preferred by the other informants included "managing a greenhouse," being "a carpenter," and working in a "warehouse." Although they did not consider their past employment histories in the community, the informants did not believe their employment aspirations were unrealistic ambitions considering their age and gender.

Three of the informants also wished to establish long-term relationships with members of the opposite sex. They felt these relationships would contribute to their sense of fulfillment in the community:

> Because I want a lasting relationship. I've seen how happy some married couples are. I've seen my brother and his girlfriend. They're married common-law. But, ah, a long-standing relationship means security for me.

> I want a nice wife, and, you know, a happy little family, you know, to raise. And, you know, be my own and that. That seems great. That's what it's all about.

These informants stated, however, that financial self-sufficiency was necessary before they could make commitments to others. The informant who felt his return to the community was a continuation of his "struggle to make it" did not seem to anticipate interpersonal relationships within the community:

> Full time job, a steady girlfriend, some leisure activities. I think that would make for a healthy lifestyle . . . um, just the everyday things.

> I'm gonna make a promise to myself that I'm gonna get out of that group home in ____, and get an apartment. And earn a . . . wage and eventually, eventually get back on my own and eventually earn my own keep, you know.

> Just going to school and getting a good education so I can get a good job, and so, you know, I can eventually get a girlfriend and settle down and have a family, you know. Work to live. . . . So that's what I want out of life. That's what I'm working towards. Yeah, I'll get it someday.

The informants' long-term aspiration was to become *ordinary*. In his last interview one of the informants confirmed that his aspiration was to become *ordinary*:

I: To be as ordinary as possible. [pause] Like mother wanted me to go into law, but, ah, law and politics. I don't think I'll ever be able to do that now. I'm too scandalous.

R: As ordinary as possible. In what sort of ways?

I: As far as holding down a job. [pause] Ah, [pause] just holding a normal job, leading a normal life. Going to the movies once a week. Taking a girlfriend out for dinner. Cleaning house.

The informants did not anticipate instant fulfillment of their aspirations and as a result all of them had strategies for gaining entry into the community.

Gaining Entry to the Community

Before leaving the hospital the informants in this study recognized their need for living accommodation and for financial support in the community. Securing living accommodations was a concern for these informants as they anticipated being unable to return to previous residential arrangements. Although the informants desired independent living in the distant future, this was not an immediate posthospitalization preference. Most of the informants initially anticipated placement in alternative living arrangements (approved or group homes) within the community. One informant anticipated living with family members. The informants sought shared accommodations because they recognized their need for companionship and support in the community:

Ah, this time I feel I'll be stronger and more capable of dealing with it, especially with living in a group home situation. I'll have support there . . . you have somebody to talk to after the day and reveal your problems to.

The informant who planned to reside with family members said that independent accommodation "seemed kind of lonely, I guess. I don't know if I could handle it."

The informants who requested referrals to alternative community placements felt they had a choice regarding these placements. For example, one informant said procurement of an alternative community placement would hasten his attending physician's decision to discharge him:

> They [alternative living arrangements] are the easiest and quickest way to get discharged. . . . Well as long as you have a place to live, you get a discharge. As long as someone is willing to take responsibility for you.

When asked about independent living accommodations, he said, "I'd probably get a place and be discharged, [but] I feel an approved home is the best situation for me right now."

This freedom of choice, however, was limited by the informants' reluctance to enter into independent living arrangements and they usually agreed to the first available placement that accepted them regardless of their assessment of the appropriateness of the placement:

> Temporary, I don't want to live there very long. If I'm there for a year, I'm . . . it's gonna be a miracle 'cause I know darn well the people of ____ don't—aren't—isn't—aren't, they're not ready for me, and I'm not ready for them.

> It's a different situation, um, it's not an easy one to do, you know. Especially like . . . I don't really like her. [laugh] To tell you the truth, to tell you the truth, I don't really like her, and I don't like the way she does things. But it's my only home for right now, so I'm just gonna, you know, do the best I can, and you know, try to, try to make it work, you know, and everything.

Both of these informants, however, intended to be discharged to these community placements.

Only one of the four informants obtained accommodation in his preferred community placement. This was the informant who planned to live with family members. The plans of the other informants failed to materialize after the community agencies rejected them as candidates for placement. Consequently, two of the three informants decided to seek independent living accommodations within their preadmission communities:

> Well, I figured the group homes weren't available to me and the approved homes weren't available for me in the ____ area. The next best thing to do was get a place of my own.

> She's been feeling a little bit sick, so she didn't really need the extra stress on her, or anything like that. So, um, she just said that she couldn't take

me and that . . . I'm ready to find my own place. Like, I wanna go to school
and stuff like that, you know. I don't wanna be sitting in here any longer.

At the time this study was completed, the fourth informant remained
in the hospital.

The second immediate concern for the informants was the ar-
rangement of financial support. All of the informants aspired to
achieve financial independence in the distant future; however, immediate financial support was required in order for them to be
discharged. This financial support was arranged by the hospital's
social services department. Although the informants expressed satisfaction with the available financial support, they felt this support
was temporary assistance.

Anchoring Future Aspirations

The informants wanted to be independent, productive members
of their community. In addition to securing accommodation and
financial support, the informants who *anticipated mastery* of their
community environments formulated plans of action oriented toward attaining their goals. The informant who did not feel entry into
the community was an opportunity to start over did not formulate
any plans beyond attaining community placement.

The informants who felt their entry into the community constituted
"starting a new life" had strategies for achieving their future goals.
The intended outcome of these plans was to establish themselves in
the community, culminating in the achievement of financial self-sufficiency. Because the informants felt financial self-sufficiency was
necessary before they could make any romantic commitments, their
primary focus was on finding employment.

These informants understood the influence of community factors
on employment opportunities, and they anticipated retaining supplementary financial support until paid employment was obtained:

I'll, I'll try to find a job. If I can't find a job, I'll live off social assistance
awhile until I can go to school.

Um, Canada Pension said that if I couldn't work they would pay me four
hundred dollars a month, and I figure that's fair. If I can't work at least I
won't starve or put anyone out.

Two of the informants anticipated rapid transition to productive roles in the competitive marketplace. Both of these informants initiated their plans for procuring employment in the community prior to discharge. The first informant contacted family members regarding employment opportunities in his community. The second informant, who wanted to become a nurse, planned to enroll in high school upgrading courses offered at a community college, and he obtained a college application form during a leave of absence from the hospital.

The third informant did not anticipate immediate employment in the competitive marketplace. Because he felt he needed a slower transition he sought self-satisfaction in the community through less competitive means. He was the only informant in this study who purposefully planned to attend community-based treatment programs. This informant believed such treatment programs would help him achieve self-reliance:

> I don't know if it's life skills, or whatever it's called. It'll be psychotherapy in one degree or another, and rehab in another. [To put me] in a position to be able to go back to work again. . . . In a month from now, I should be on AISCH [disability pension], working part time, attending programs, getting back into society on an even basis, or a controlled basis rather.

If unable to obtain part-time employment this informant said he might volunteer to work with the Canadian Mental Health Association as an alternative means of contributing to the community.

All of the informants anticipated contact with health care professionals in the community. Only one informant felt these professionals would help him adjust to community life. The other two informants felt that community-based professionals would only be helpful for follow-up drug therapy. Neither of these informants expressed unconditional acceptance of the continued need for drug therapy in the community.

The first of these two informants compared mental health care to quicksand:

> Well, you're not ever gonna get away from it. . . . Like, I'll have to go home, and I'll have to take medication for the rest of my life.

Although this informant reluctantly accepted his need for continued drug therapy in his interviews, he denied his need for drug therapy in his statements to a family member. The family member told the researcher that this informant had suggested he may discontinue his medications after discharge. When this relative informed him that compliance with his drug therapy was a condition of his accommodation he consented to comply with continued drug therapy. The second informant planned to seek professional assistance in undertaking a drug-free trial in the community:

> Like, when I get to ____, I'm gonna see a doctor, and I'm gonna gradually take myself off this, and see how I do, you know.

The informant who felt he was not ready to return to the community did not describe strategies for achieving his future goals. Beyond obtaining community placement, this informant was uncertain about his future plans:

> I don't know. . . . If I can't find something to do, I might have to leave it. . . . Well, I go into the group home on December the first, I guess. They promised me that, go into the group home on December the first. So I got that, but then I, I don't know how I'll manage after that.

Furthermore, this informant recognized his inability to formulate concrete plans for the future. For example, beyond his inability to obtain employment he could not identify a reason for his jobless status:

> I don't think there is. . . . I'm gonna go out and earn it. So I just don't know how to go about it. I need guidance . . . [from] people, myself, things around me.

This informant also recognized his need for further rehabilitation in the community, but his references to community-based treatment were uncertain. He did not establish either explicit time lines or anticipated behavioral outcomes he hoped to achieve by attending community-based programs:

Well, I'd probably have to be a whole bunch of rehabilitation somewhere. And that's maybe what I'm must sort of entering into. Maybe I should take . . . that daycare program up at the hospital in ____. Well, I'm gonna have to do something in ____, so maybe that'd be a good start.

Although all the informants in this study wanted to become self-supporting community members, apart from strategies associated with gaining entry into the community one informant did not formulate concrete plans for attaining his long-term goals. This informant did not feel he was ready to return to the community and as a result he was unsure about his future plans.

Expressing Positive Self-Regard

The third indicator of *anticipating mastery* was expressing a positive self-regard. The self-references made by the informants in this study varied as much as their assessments of their readiness to return to the community. Those respondents who felt they were ready for discharge expressed positive self-regard. These informants said their present mental well-being had improved in comparison to their preadmission well-being:

I just feel better about myself. I'm able to breathe properly. I've got a song in my heart, a whistle on my lips.

I feel really good about myself. I like myself a lot.

Although the third informant did not make direct self-references, he described himself as feeling less "bogged down" and "discouraged": "Well, I kind of hope I'm never in this . . . get bogged down and as bad shape as when I started anyway."

In contrast, the informant who felt he was not ready to return to the community made disparaging self-references:

I'm, I'm just a creep, you know. I'm just a creep in sheep's clothing. . . . I'm just afraid whether you'll think I'm a joke or something—as some kind of a last joke going on in the universe or something really stupid. . . . My mind is so small, you know. Sometimes I feel like I don't even have a mind.

This informant also described himself as "degenerating" and "pretty screwed up," and he did not identify any changes in his mental well-being since his admission to hospital:

> You know, I'm, ah, I'm pretty screwed up, man. But later on maybe I'll get it together. But [pause] it's still the same. I'm, I'm a human being, right? . . . I just hate the thoughts going [on] in my head.

Moreover, he consistently said that his mental well-being had deteriorated since his first contact with mental health professionals:

> I started to do stupid things at home so my father figured I needed help, and I probably did. But I don't know what kind of help it was. It didn't seem to help too much. . . . When I went there the first time, it never [worked] so . . . look at where I am now. I'm worse off than I was when I went in there. I would have been better off just to stay the hell away! . . . But I, I don't think I'll ever be the same as I was when I was growing up. I don't know how it happened. I just got involved. I got the first series of treatment, and then, and then I just never recovered, you know.

The variance in the informants' self-regard was also reflected in their feelings of self-confidence. One informant described self-confidence as:

> being able to walk into a place with my head up. Being able to sit down and be pleasant and bright; order a meal without any hassles within myself.

The informants who felt they were ready to return to the community expressed self-confidence:

> Oh, I admit I have problems, it's just that I've learned how to deal with them.

> I've got the brains and stamina enough to, um, take advantage of this and make something out of my life.

The informant who believed he was not ready to return to the community described his present abilities as inadequate: "It's only manual dexterity and skills . . . that if I had more accomplishment and more know how, I wouldn't be in trouble." In addition, this informant continued to express feelings of being overwhelmed:

> Somethings, somethings make it—somethings will start me up and then shut me down, eh, in this hospital. It's very unreal. Sometimes I feel better than others, and then automatically I'll switch back to a bad mood.

He also characterized himself as "decentered":

> I don't have any problem, you see. I don't happen to have a center of gravity there, that's all. I go tumbling down the hill all the time.

This informant's lack of self-autonomy precluded feelings of self-confidence.

The informants in this study who felt they were ready for discharge expressed feelings of positive self-regard and self-reliance. In contrast, the informant who did not believe he was ready to return to the community was self-depreciating and he continued to describe himself as being overwhelmed.

Gaining Control of Intrusive Experiences

Two informants described gaining control of the effects of intrusive experiences on their behaviors. As a result, they experienced unique changes in their well-being. Also, disagreements with hospital professionals regarding their readiness for discharge based on the presence of these experiences resulted in these informants assuming a more assertive stance when seeking discharge.

The particular control behaviors initiated by these two informants were derived from their perception of the nature of the intrusive experiences. The informants did not absolutely accept the professionals' contention that these experiences were intrapsychic phenomena:

> It's true, let me tell you. As God is my witness. I believe it's because I . . . hear voices, and I know for sure that it's true because they can read my thoughts. Like I have someone right now even reading my thoughts.

The other informant said what he hears is "real":

I: I figure I don't hallucinate it half as much as what I hear.
R: Yeah, you've told me that before—what you hear is real.
I: Generally. I'll grant some of what I hear . . . is garbled, is misinterpreted by me. But if I misinterpret something, I generally ask the question "Why" or "What" or "Did you say that."

The failure of psychotropic drugs to eradicate these experiences was interpreted by these informants as substantiating their contention that these experiences were objectively real:

R: And that's when they tried you on that new drug?
I: Yeah, yeah, but it didn't work, you know. I mean, if there's a transmitter in your room, I mean, no matter I was on 900 milligrams of chlorpromazine a day, and I was still hearing voices. So that must tell you something. I could be on 1800 milligrams of chlorpromazine a day, and I could still hear voices if they're there. Lately, they haven't been there.
R: But if they're there, they're there.
I: They're there, they're there. No drug's gonna—I know what I hear. I know what I see.

The second informant also had similar beliefs:

> With this medication, the super drugs they put me on, and the heavy doses they put me on, I shouldn't hallucinate. . . . Actually, I didn't tell them that. I—the thought just came to me. I'm gonna use it the next time they tell me I'm hallucinating. Usually, I just kept my mouth shut and grin and bear it.

These informants attempted to identify the external sources of these auditory stimuli. One of them maintained that his proclaimed source is indisputable:

> She believed that I hear voices, but she didn't believe there was a transmitter in my room, you know. And, of course, there is, you know. It might not be inside my room, but it's, it's just outside my room possibly, you know. And I hear these voices. That's it.

The second informant was not as certain about the source of these experiences. He said some of his auditory stimuli *may be* hallucinations. He defined hallucinations as "hearing things that aren't there." Distinguishing between objectively-based auditory stimuli and hallucinations, however, was difficult for this informant. An experience was classified as a hallucination only after all possible sources of environmental causation were eliminated:

> As in where I am, where I am in relation to the room. What I'm picking up could be conversations down the hall. It's echoing, or it could be something coming through the air vent that's shares with, like the nursing offices. There's an air vent that comes down, and I can sometimes hearing them talking in there. . . . Then if I can't, if I can't analyze it scientifically and decide, if I can't give it a feasible reason where it's coming from, then I decide it's a hallucination.

Nevertheless, this informant accounted for the intrusive experiences by referring to a broad range of potential environmental sources:

> Well, lately it's been—I've been called a child abuser, a faggot. . . . Staff do it to stress me out and see if I can take it or not. Patients do it just to be downright nasty. They want some sort of power over each other. . . . It's like a pecking order in a hen house. . . . Oh, [pause] one of the games like "Wear my face" or [pause] something like that or stuff like that. . . . If you look at somebody and they don't like the way you look at them, they'll say, "Wear my face." . . . It means you're suppose to hallucinate and think that you're wearing their face. This is a reminder that you are not suppose to look them in the eye. . . . Yeah, it's hypnosis is all it is. Suggestion and feeling suggestions, and—I don't know. Half of the hallucinations I ever got in my life are due to hypnosis.

When this informant was not experiencing or discussing probable intrusive experiences he was able to relate to these experiences as if they were hallucinations:

> I: If I have an overload of information, I hallucinate. Uh, [pause] that's about it, and when that happens, I get frustrated and angry, and I get paranoid. . . . I kept hearing other conversations and figured they were talking about me.
> R: During that, do you realize what's going on?
> I: I do now.

When this informant was experiencing these sensations during the interviews or was discussing probable intrusive experiences, however, he related to them as if they were objectively real experiences. For example, he was frequently distracted during the interviews. He would occasionally turn his head aside and mutter profanities. He attributed the cause of his distraction to environmental stimuli such as voices in a passing car.

Regardless of the attributed source of these experiences both of these informants described gaining some control over the behavioral effects of the experiences. The methods they used to gain control may be classified as proactive and reactive behaviors. Proactive behaviors were behaviors initiated by the informants in order to affect the quality/quantity of the incoming stimuli. In contrast, the intent of reactive behaviors was to modify the informants' response to the incoming stimuli.

Proactive Strategies

Modification of the quality and/or the quantity of incoming auditory stimuli was achieved by enacting behaviors designed to alter one of two aspects of the intrusive experience. The first type of proactive behaviors were behaviors directed toward the perceived source of the stimuli. One informant described confronting the perceived source in order to suppress further intrusions:

> I was taking my meds, minding my own business, and another guy was talking while I was distracted. And then all of the sudden he starts calling me "Faggot! You fairy! Everybody hates you!" and this and that and started walking away. And I yelled out his name, right, very loudly. And he turned around and says "Ah, you faggot, fairy! You coward!" I blew up, just went into a rage. . . . I jumped him. I pushed him down actually.

Proactive behaviors directed toward the perceived source of the auditory stimuli were not necessarily aggressive behaviors. The second informant described using his "voices" as mediators in order to bargain with the perceived source of the intrusive experiences:

I: I'm still trying to get them to tell me that she'll have coffee with me, but I can't convince them. [laugh]
R: You can't convince them yet?
I: No, I try, try everything, I'm telling you, I do.

As well as attempting to contact the perceived source through his "voices," this informant also endeavored to establish contact through associates of the perceived source living in the community:

> And she just wrote me a letter back and just told me everything was okay, you know. Everything was—"Hey, you never did that much to our family." And, you know, "We forgive you for anything that you might of done." And all that, so, you know, everything is okay.

It should be noted that the content of these informants' intrusive experiences were markedly different. The "voices" of the first informant were punitive, while the "voices" of the second participant were positive and nonthreatening.

The second type of proactive behaviors involved deflecting incoming stimuli by directing attention away from the intrusive "voices." These behaviors were implemented by the informant who heard punitive "voices." Redirection strategies included concentrating on conversations with others and concentrating on bodily movements:

> I was a little stressed out in the restaurant tonight. You were there, and you were talking to me, so I didn't feel too bad. . . . So I just kept listening to my mouth chewing and listening to you, and I felt okay.

Reactive Strategies

The intent of reactive behaviors was to alter personal responses to auditory stimuli. Reactive behaviors consisted of both passive and active behaviors. Both informants described passively ignoring auditory stimuli:

> I don't let certain things bother me anymore. By certain things I mean just small problems that arose in day-to-day life living in an institution. . . . Ah, I would say people stealing things spiritually [pause] or giving things spiritually. Things that can't be seen . . . because I feel that as long as I'm breathing and thinking that I don't have to worry about spiritual things anymore. And it's—if they're there, they're there. And if they're not, they're gone.

I know that they're lies. I know that they're lies. They're not, they're not truth. They lie, so I just don't believe them. . . . I just don't believe everything I hear these days. I use to believe in everything I was told, eh?

The informant who heard punitive "voices" described implementing active-reactive behaviors. These were purposeful behaviors designed to reduce this informant's feelings of anger and tension:

I sigh and relax. Make yourself be nonviolent. Make yourself be as calm as possible. . . . Then it's a fantasy, and then I resolve that and say, "That was a fantasy, and I'm not going to listen to it anymore, and it's not there" and go on to something different. . . . With me it goes away. Sometimes it takes a little work. Sometimes I have to go take a bath or a long walk or just go to sleep and forget about it.

This informant felt the psychotropic medications were an adjunct to his reactive strategies:

It's, ah, a matter of over abundance of stimulus or stimuli—I hallucinate. Where with the neuroleptic drugs, the tranquilizers, or neuroleptic would be a major tranquilizer, I don't freak out about it anymore. It comes and passes. . . . I feel sedated but not restrained. [pause] Uh, the violence in me is restrained, but the rest, the freedom of thought isn't.

Although he said the medications alleviated his feelings of depression, the informant who described his present intrusive experiences as nonthreatening did not think medications affected those experiences or his immediate reaction to them:

Now I feel, I feel lots better. This flupenthixol is a miracle drug. It is! It is! Who ever invented it, I'd like to write them a letter and tell them "Thank you for helping me." I really would because it's, it's so good that I feel, I feel so much better. It's—it had an antidepressant effect on ya and, um, it's so much better.

Gaining control over the effects of these experiences contributed to these informants' improved sense of well-being. Prior to gaining this control these informants characterized the intrusions as repressive. In order to protect their well-being they reacted either through acting out or withdrawing. Gaining control of these experiences reduced their repressive effects allowing them to direct their attention to other aspects of their environment.

The informants' predischarge descriptions of the effects of intrusive experiences on their personal well-being were antipodal to those recollected during the preadmission period. One of the informants recalled being "preoccupied" and "mentally restricted" as a consequence of these experiences. At predischarge he described himself as emancipated from these effects:

> You know, they don't, they don't interfere with my, you know, they don't preoccupy me too much, you know. They don't interfere with my daily routines and stuff like that. . . . I can go out and do the things that I want to now. And before, I was basically restricted mentally, you know.

The other informant recalled being "distracted" and "frustrated" by these experiences. He described himself as being in a "cold rage." During the predischarge period he said this rage had dissipated: "I'm much more calm, my head is clearer. . . . I don't feel the inner turmoil that I use to." He also stated he was less distracted: "I'm able to read and write again. I'm able to listen to television and radio again."

These two informants rejected the professionals' contentions that their experiences were intrapsychic phenomena and they also rejected the idea that these experiences implied mental illness. They felt their experiences were unique because they or the source of the intrusions possessed exceptional characteristics. For example, during one interview one of the informants asked the interviewer if she heard a voice call him "murderer." He said her failure to hear this voice was due to her less "acute" hearing. The second informant said his experiences were unique because the source had an exceptional ability: "She hired a person that has this special gift to read my mind." Basically, these two informants felt they were psychologically ordinary people who had extraordinary experiences.

The Hospital Experience: Being in a "Boot Camp"

One informant said being in hospital is analogous to being in an army "boot camp." He based his comparison on the similarities between the structures and the functions of these organizations. In much the same way as a boot camp, the hospital segregates patients from the pedestrian community, is a temporary situation designed to prepare patients for community living, is a residential facility established and managed by service providers for service recipients, is a receptacle for "conscripted" service recipients, and is an institution in which interpersonal relationships are based on "expert authoritarianism":

> It's like entering boot camp in the army. . . . It's an exercise in discipline for yourself, the staff, from the staff. You have to be good. . . . When you are able to accept discipline from somebody that's in a position to give it to you and have discipline for yourself, take care of yourself, that's when you're ready to leave.

Although the other informants in this study did not make this analogy, their interviews confirmed the appropriateness of this comparison.

Being in a Boot Camp

Segregating Patients from the Pedestrian Community

The informants in this study perceived the hospital as an institution detached from the community. They described their admission in terms of being "sent away" from their preadmission communities:

> He just sent me straight up here.

> We're shipping you to ____.

In contrast, leaving the hospital was referred to as "reentering" the community:

> It's a reentry into society.

> It'll mean I'm finally accepted back into society.

Furthermore, the informants felt the hospital was detached from its surrounding community: "Well, you're a few miles from any civilization. It's extremely quiet outside." Excursions into the neighboring town were referred to as going "up to town" or "going into the town."

Leaves of absence from the hospital were sanctioned excursions into the pedestrian community. The informants characterized these leaves as trials to evaluate their readiness to return to the community:

> It's just that I'm feeling more adapted to it as each LOA [leave of absence] confirms.

> Ready and able to deal with myself and society.

> I was—I wasn't making no trouble at my approved home, you know. I was being in on time and going to sleep and not getting up quite when I was suppose to, but that can be worked on.

Leaves of absence were planned, temporary reintegrations into the community, although excursions into the town adjacent to the hospital were seen as recreation because they were privileges granted by the hospital's professionals:

> A couple of weeks ago I got full privileges. . . . I'm able to go to town and come back when I please. I can walk into town whenever I want to. I don't have to check in during the day. I just have to be here for meal times and med times.

Despite being outside of the geographical boundaries of the institution the informants with town privileges continued to see themselves as appendages of the hospital community.

Preparing Patients For Community Living

The belief that psychiatric hospitals are institutions for the treatment of people unable to function in the community persisted throughout the interviews in this study. During a termination interview one informant said that psychiatric care centers are for:

> people that are emotionally sick or have psychological problems or physiological problems. That means they just can't cope with society on a day-to-day level.

All of the informants felt their hospitalizations were temporary and they anticipated returning to the community in the future: "At least there's a beginning and an end to ____, anyway." According to these informants the primary function of the hospital was to resolve their personal problems and help them return to community living:

> It's, you see, it's an establishment for putting you back on your own again.

> The facility's good, you know. I'd suggest it to anyone that is having problems coping with life, and you know, you know, just to get their problems set up.

The informants in this study felt that guardianship issues should not be the primary concern of the hospital staff:

> Perhaps it's not so much of a dodge as people covering their back, covering their backdoor. Making sure when I go home I'm not a time bomb and go out and get physical. Go out and start trouble, eh?

When the informants felt guardian concerns were taking precedence over perceived treatment needs, they became angry and frustrated:

> I find it's an insult. I don't go around generally attacking people, verbally or mentally, or verbally or physically, rather.

A Residential Facility Managed by Service Providers

Recipients of psychiatric care live in a milieu created by others. Admission to a psychiatric hospital compels the individual to relinquish previous life-styles and adapt to communal institutional living and the institution's standards of expected conduct; however, the characteristics of the institutional milieu vary within the hospital. The hospital is partitioned into nursing units, each with a designated patient population. The milieu of these units varies markedly and it is contingent on the type of service provided by the unit. All of the informants in this study began their stay in the hospital on admission units and later they were transferred to rehabilitation units.

Admission Units

All of the informants had a negative view of the admission unit. They said their experience on this unit was similar to being incarcerated, that is, being "locked up":

I didn't like it at all when I was on _____, you know. It was . . . terrible, you
know. Just . . . the feeling of being locked up is just an awful feeling, you
know. I can never stand being in jail or anything like that, you know. Like,
I wouldn't do anything to go to jail or anything like that, you know. But I
don't know. . . . It was a terrible feeling. I can't even explain it, you know.
I just, it's just . . . terrible, you know, being locked up like that. Like, like
you're locked up in a cage, eh? You can't go nowhere. You can't do
anything. Sure they have pool tables, and they have ping-pong tables, and
they have juice, and they have people around to talk to, and stuff like that,
but still, it's not a good feeling to be locked up in a place like that.

The informants also said that the service providers on the admission
unit were authoritative:

The staff can be extremely domineering on the admission wards. It's
their . . . exerting their authority. And you come to know, and come to
grips with the reality of being in an institution where there are certain rules
that must be followed.

They lock you out of bed, and go along there, and hustle you in a group
all the time.

The informants also felt they were overmedicated and received
impersonal care on the admission unit:

It's a very heavy sedate ward. They sedate you like crazy on the ward, and
then they send you to another ward from there if you're not able to leave.
Well, usually the stay is quite long, eh? So you get fed up to the point
where you're kicking or hitting someone, and they send, they fire you into
another part of the hospital.

One informant said he could not recall his feelings regarding his
transfer to a rehabilitation unit:

I was pretty knocked out and wacked out, severely medicated, and I was
very confused. . . . I was just being handled like a crate.

Rehabilitation Units

The informants had both positive and negative opinions about the
rehabilitation unit, and the quality of their evaluation depended on

their standard of comparison. The informants were positive about the rehabilitation unit when they compared it to the admission units:

> Well, on ____, like that's a pretty open ward. There's a lot of freedom there. There isn't much freedom on—when I first came in here.

> The same thing only not as intense. They're more of your buddies here. Once you get better, it's sort of like, ah, after shock.

> I came over to ____, and it was even better, eh? You know, open ward. I can come and go as I please, you know. I don't have to check in at any time, you know. I can just go whenever I want to, you know, and that was great.

When the informants compared the rehabilitation unit with their previous life-style, however, they said these units were similar to "jails." Although the informants did not feel locked up, which was their main impression of the admission units, they felt the rehabilitation unit was similar to jail because it involved group living and the regulation of their behavior by others:

> I have to eat meals with a lot of people. I have to sleep in my own cubicle with other people around. I have to sit in the same room with a lot of other people. [pause] If I fist fight, I'm in trouble. [pause] If I blow my cool, I get medication . . . and I have people exerting an authority over me. I'm use to being independent and living on my own.

> Just whereas your freedoms are confined to a certain area. You have to be in at a certain time. Um, your meals are all cooked for you. You go down, stand in line like you would in jail, you know, and get your food and, you know, eat and then go back up to the ward. Take you meds, hang out for awhile, you know, make a call once in awhile, have visitors once in awhile.

> Um, just um, 'cause you're, you're restricted to a ward. You gotta be in at a certain time. Um, you have to get up in the mornings and go to work, you know. . . . I've never been to jail so I can't—I'm just saying it as a fact that, um, that it seem like to me, it's, it's a lot like what jail would be like.

A Receptacle for "Conscripted" Service Recipients

The informants in this study attributed their admission to the interventions of other people and not one informant described his admission as self-initiated. As a result they felt the hospital community was composed of two broad groups of people: "insiders" and "outsiders." From the informants' perspective, service recipients are the insiders and service providers are the outsiders of the institution. Insiders are totally immersed in the institutional milieu; whereas outsiders, in addition to creating the milieu, are detached from it:

> The way they give their treatment . . . it's based on real society. [pause]. . . . On being on the outside. How an outside person would deal with you. After all, they are from the outside. Living, working on the inside. We have to live it, but they work it.

Once they were admitted to the hospital the informants became members of the insiders group; however, this mandatory group assignment was not favored by the informants as none of them wanted to be associated with the insider group:

> You have to come back [from leaves of absence (LOAs)] and sit around with sick people again and listen to them cry and whine. You know, I suppose, I suppose, I suppose it's to evoke some compassion in a person, but to live with it, day in and day out, gets kind of tiring.

> What am I doing here? You know, there's all these sick people around me and, you know, I'm totally sane, you know. There's nothing wrong with me. How am I suppose to feel?

Another informant told the researcher that the other study participants were "crackpots." Usually, when the informants did make references to peer relationships with other patients, they described these patients as not "sick."

The informants in this study wanted to be associated with the outsider group, and because they felt the members of the nursing staff were exemplars of this group the informants aspired to emulate their qualities: "Something like the people here in this hospital. Like the . . . nurses and stuff. You know what I mean." One informant said his desire to become a nurse was a result of his experiences with the hospital's nurses:

> I just met a lot of nice nurses and stuff like that, and I like the job that they do and everything like that. That's what I'd like to be doing myself, eh?

A third informant explicitly rejected affiliation with the insider group. He described the nursing professionals as his "peers":

> Talking to the staff is, because they're educated. I've got a certain amount of education myself. . . . To me, they're my peers unless, unless the patients have been to school and studied. It's just not the same.

An Institution in Which Relationships Are Based on "Expert Authoritarianism"

Expert authoritarianism refers to relationships that are characterized by obedience to experts and this term describes four recurring themes in the data associated with the relationship between the hospital's professionals and the informants: institutional privileges and community resources were accessed through the professionals; the decision to "promote" patients was the prerogative of experts; experts' assessments of readiness for "promotion" were valued by the informants; and the informants complied with aspects of their treatment they considered nontherapeutic.

Institutional Privileges and Community Resources

At admission the hospital's professionals imposed constraints on the informants' freedom of movement. Personal liberties were incrementally regained as professionals granted the informants privileges, which were described as having three levels. The first level, "close watch," required that the informant was accompanied by staff members when leaving the unit. When limited privileges were granted the informant was "allowed to go out for a few hours at a time, not up to town, but to stay on the hospital's grounds." Acquisition of full privileges allowed the informants to leave the hospital's grounds; however, they were required to return to their units for meals and medications. One informant who had full privileges described himself as a "trustee": "Well, now that I'm a trustee, it's not too bad."

Community resources were also accessed through professionals. The type of formal community assistance sought by informants in this study depended on their personal resources in the community. For example, in order to leave the hospital supplementary financial support was required by all the informants. This financial support was arranged by the hospital's social services department and the informants said they had no difficulties accessing this support:

> I kept on him [social worker] by asking him about getting out and making arrangements to get my AISCH [pension] reinstated and things like that. So he went down with me a week ago Thursday, a week ago today, and we got the ball rolling for paper work on my AISCH.

The second type of formal community assistance sought by the informants was alternative community placements. Three of the informants required these placements because they were unable to return to their previous living accommodations. In order for these informants to obtain these placements two groups of experts had to approve the informants' candidacy: hospital professionals and community placement operators.

The hospital's professionals referred the informants to community placements. As previously indicated, the informants had a choice regarding placement in alternative living arrangements; however, access to the hospital's social workers was limited because of these professionals' caseloads:

> We tried various placement programs, and seeing as the social worker is dealing with thirty to sixty other people at the same time, I have to wait my turn.

Once the informant was approved for community placement the operators of these community residences assessed the informant's suitability for placement. Although the hospital's professionals assessed the informants' readiness for placement, frequently the community placement professionals did not concur with their assessments. Two of the informants were rejected as placement candidates; the third informant was conditionally accepted. One informant who was rejected was advised by the community placement operators to reapply for placement in one month:

> They said come back in a month. We're not turning you down permanently. We just feel that you are not ready yet, and we want you to come back in a month and reapply.

The operators of another community residence imposed conditions on the informant before they would accept him:

> I, ah, I'm happy to go there, but I wasn't, I didn't want to go on their arrangements. They wanted me to come there in a matter of three or four [four LOAs] and at the first of December move in.

The Decision to Promote Patients Was the Prerogative of Experts

The informants' discharge from the hospital depended on their attending physicians; consequently, the act of discharge was an action performed by others:

> Actually if they said a few days and that was a week ago, it should have been a couple of days ago. . . . I don't think they're in any rush to let me go.

> Just the fact that she [physician] wouldn't, you know, she wouldn't let me go, or nothing like that, you know. She wouldn't, she was being obstinate with me and stuff like that. Especially after I saw that other doctor, um, you know. She . . . really wanted me to stick around for awhile.

> Every time I say within two to three weeks, it ends up being a month later. So . . . I believe them when they come up to me one day and say, "____, pack your bags. We're going to ____."

> It's like the donkey and the carrot. Holding the discharge in front of my nose, and then, the last minute snatching it away.

All of the informants in this study were voluntary patients, and they were aware of their legal right to leave the hospital:

> And now that I got the voluntary status, I know that I have the choice to leave. I can leave.

> Of course, I could, I could leave right now. I could just pack my things and say, "I'm going." There's nothing they could do about it.

Although limited personal resources prohibited the informants from discharging themselves against medical advice, even when alternative community resources were obtained, they still sought a professional discharge. The informants' desire for a professional promotion was related to their perception of the professionals' area of expertise.

Experts' Assessment of Readiness for Promotion

The hospital's experts evaluated the informants' mental well-being and formed authoritative judgments regarding their readiness to return to the community:

> Well, the doctor, Dr. ____, didn't believe me. She . . . believed that I was still too sick to go out into the community.

> They've decided that I'm more coherent in my speech. I'm not deluded, or I have very few delusions. Things that aren't gonna make me incompatible with the people around me or on the outside.

Also, it was important to the informants who assessed themselves ready to return to the community to obtain professional approval:

> By going through, going through the ropes, to use a cliché, I feel more comfortable having the approval of somebody professional saying, "Yes ____, you're ready to leave."

For these informants, professional consent to leave the hospital represented professional confirmation of their sanity:

> It will mean that I am certifiably sane . . . and I can say to somebody, if somebody says to me, "Ah, you're crazy," I can say, "No, I'm not. I've got a piece of paper to prove it."

> Well, that's a good feeling [to get discharged]. At least you know you're half sane anyway. . . . Well, [pause], you never know. There could be something wrong, like you watch on TV all the time.

The informant who felt he was not ready to return to the community was uncertain about the meaning of being discharged from hospital. When asked what discharge meant to him, he said, "I don't know. I'm not around any of my relatives."

*Participants Were Compliant with Treatment They Considered
Nontherapeutic*

The informants said they complied with all aspects of their hospital
care, regardless of the perceived therapeutic value of specific interventions. They complied with therapies they considered nontherapeutic because of their subordinate position within the organization
and the accompanying dependency on the benevolence of experts:

> They told me, they told me the shots that were being taken. So I just . . .
> agreed with that and went peacefully, you know. I wasn't gonna put up
> too much of a fight, you know. . . . I could have, you know. I could have
> really raised hell, you know, around here, but there's no use in it, you
> know. There's no satisfaction out of it, you know. I don't get nothing out
> of it for raising hell, so I'll . . . just do what they tell me to do, you know.
> For once in my life, I'll listen to somebody, you know, rather than doing
> my own thing, you know. Yeah. . . . Ah, it would get me nowhere. It would
> just upset things, you know. Screw up the whole system and, you know,
> it's . . . not worth it.

One informant said he attended structured therapy sessions he
perceived as nontherapeutic because "if I wanna get a place in the
group home or approved home, I have to go through this course."
Two of the informants felt their vocational programs had no therapeutic value, and compliance with authoritative directives accounted for their attendance:

> They send you to OT [occupational therapy] for one hour a day, you know,
> and you're suppose to work and stuff like that, you know. But I just . . .
> find little use in it, you know. I . . . don't like it. Maybe I'm a rebel. I don't
> know, but I don't like it one bit.

Only one informant felt his vocational program had any therapeutic
value. He did not, however, believe these programs helped him
develop work skills; instead, he felt they provided an environment
for testing his ability to manage stressful situations:

> When I started working in the snack bar, I felt more competent about being
> around more other people, and being—putting myself in a social situation
> where the noise level and the conversation level was quite high—the
> potential for getting strained.

Although the informants in this study disliked institutional living, their overall evaluation of their hospital experience was not negative. The informants who had previous admissions to the institution were neutral about their hospital experience: "Oh well, it's not too bad [to be here]. I can think of worse places." Although one informant said his hospitalization had not helped him recover his mental well-being, he felt his treatment was exemplary:

> I can't . . . see any better way than doing it than the way they are doing it. Just exactly the way they are doing it. 'Cause they're coming as close as I think they'll ever come to problem solving. As far as I am concerned.

The two informants who experienced their first admission to the hospital evaluated their overall experience positively. In comparison to the treatment they received in community hospitals, both of these informants said the professionals were "caring," and the hospital offered the "best" treatment in Alberta:

> If you're sick and you need treatment, it's probably the best in Alberta or in western Canada. I'd say Alberta for sure seeing as I've been in a few hospitals around. If you want treatment, it's good for a certain amount of time.

From the informants' perspective, the primary function of the hospital was to ameliorate personal problems that hinder their functioning in the community; therefore, discharge was sought when the informants felt they were ready to return to the community or when they thought the treatment provided in the hospital was not helping them return to the community.

Pathways to Discharge: "Getting Out"

The informants in this study felt that discharge from the hospital was granted by the experts and they described three patterns of discharge behaviors: marking time, taking charge, and breaking out. The particular pattern of behavior demonstrated by the informants was contingent on two factors: self-assessment of readiness to return to the community and self-assessment of the likelihood of being

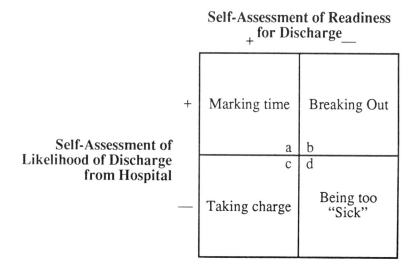

Figure 4.2. Pathways to Discharge: Patterns of Predischarge Behavior

discharged. Figure 4.2 illustrates the interaction between these conditions. Each of the four cells in the diagram describes constellations of behaviors displayed by the informants in this study. As the conditions determining the behavioral pattern vary, there is an accompanying change in the "getting out" behavior. If there is variation in the conditions affecting his discharge, one informant can be classified as fitting into more than one cell.

Marking Time

For the informants in this study, marking time meant enduring continued hospitalization: "I'll . . . make the best of it. I'll just do my thing, and just wait. I'm just doing time right now." This pattern of behavior was present when the informants felt they were ready to return to the community and when they felt there was a good chance of being discharged. The informants attributed marking time to the lack of available alternatives in the community, and they characterized their predischarge behavior as "doing time."

*Attributing Inpatient Status to a Lack
of Available Alternatives*

The informants who were marking time felt they were ready to
return to the community, and they said their continued inpatient
status was a result of their lack of personal resources necessary for
community living:

> I feel like, you know, I don't have any other place to go right now, so you
> know, it's . . . peaches and cream as far as I'm concerned, you know,
> for . . . the time being.

> Ah, [pause] I'm in a hurry if they got some money that I can live on. . . . I
> don't have anything to live on unless they are going to give me a pension.

*Characterizing Predischarge Behavior
as "Doing Time"*

When the informants exhibited marking time behavior they felt
their continued hospitalization was nontherapeutic because they
had regained their mental well-being. From this perspective the
informants considered the hospital a temporary accommodation
until they could obtain a community placement:

> I feel it in my soul, you know. I don't need to stay here any longer. I'm
> just bumming off the government right now, you know, waiting so. . . .
> It's a joke. It's a total joke. I . . . there's nothing more that they can do for
> me, you know. Like, I'm just doing time, that's all I'm doing.

> I'm just waiting for placement.

Also, the informants felt bored and frustrated waiting for community
placement:

> I've been waiting for almost two months, I'd say. So . . . it gets rather
> impatient, you know. I get bored to tears sometimes here, you know. But
> I just try to look for things to do and go down to the snack bar and have
> coffee and stuff like that when I can. And see girls and socialize a bit, and
> that's about it.

> I've been waiting for placement for the last two and a half months. . . . It's
> frustrating. It's like waiting for a big pay-off in a lottery.

Breaking Out

The informants said breaking out of hospital was returning prematurely to the community: "I wanted to get the hell out of this hospital. That's what I want." This pattern of "getting out" behavior occurred when the informants felt they were not ready to return to the community and had a good chance of getting discharged. Although this situation seems improbable, the informants did discuss this behavioral pattern. The breaking out behavior occurred when the informants felt their treatment was futile, and when this happened they had an impulsive desire to leave the hospital.

Characterizing Continued Inpatient Status as Futile in Terms of Expected Outcome

The informants who manifested breaking out behaviors felt that they were not ready to return to the community and that their treatment was not helping them recover their mental well-being:

I have to get hold of my folks and tell them that I'm coming up that way and then head, maybe head west. Because, um . . . I can't seem to get it together here.

I get very terrified as you can notice. Unless that's what basically I am. I'm just terrified of this place. . . . I'm terrified of what it can do to me and where it can take me. . . . Um, the fact that it's . . . gonna take me nowhere.

Impulsively Proposing to Leave the Hospital

The informants who had an impulsive desire to leave the hospital said their present hospital stay was nontherapeutic. The rationale for this judgment was their perception that their treatment was not improving their mental well-being; therefore, the primary reason for seeking discharge was to get away from the hospital. These informants impulsively proposed leaving the hospital without considering their expected proficiency in managing in the community or the availability of placement:

The more I think about it, the more I think I should just pack up and leave right now.

Yeah, we should take off tonight, and just go there for awhile.

I have to get a hold of my folks and tell that I'm coming up that way and then head, maybe head west.

Taking Charge

When the informants displayed taking charge behavior, they were demonstrating their readiness to leave hospital:

When I first got turn[ed] down for the group home, and then it became a real battle. . . . Well, I had to prove myself that I was ready to be discharged. And, ah, [pause] that's about it. I just had to prove that I was ready, capable of surviving on my own.

This pattern of "getting out" behavior was evident when the informants assessed themselves ready for discharge and felt there was little chance of being discharged. The informants attributed taking charge behavior to the professionals' unwillingness to authorize their discharge, and they characterized this behavior as convincing professionals of their readiness to be discharged.

Attributing Present Inpatient Status to Professionals' Unwillingness to Authorize Discharge

The informants who exhibited taking charge behavior felt they were ready to return to the community. They attributed their present hospitalization to the professionals' refusal to discharge them:

I felt that they were just playing games and trying to keep me in here as long as possible. . . . I think they are just grasping at straws to keep me in here.

I felt pissed off because she's [physician] looking at me as if I'm sick and I have a psychiatric problem, and I don't. I'm totally sane. . . . I swear to God on my mother's grave. I'm totally sane. There's nothing wrong with me, not a thing. There's no reason why I should stay here any longer.

Characterizing Behavior as "Convincing" Professionals of Readiness for Discharge

The basis for the difference between the informants' and the professionals' assessments of the informants' readiness for discharge centered on disagreement regarding the criteria for assessment. The informants felt that their readiness to leave the hospital should be evaluated on the basis of continued evidence of the behaviors that precipitated their admissions, regardless of the presence or absence of other abnormal symptoms:

> I'm not gonna OD, that's, it's not the point of the voices. It's the point of, of me ODing all the time and taking too many drugs, and stuff like that. And I'm not gonna do that no more because I feel good. There's no reason why.

> Ah, probably on my admission file, there's some strange things about my sexual nature and . . . what I was hearing at the time. [pause] I was hypnotized. . . . They're holding it against me.

Because the informants believed the major problem behaviors had been eradicated, they felt they were ready for discharge.

In order to institute behaviors intended to convince professionals of their readiness for discharge, the informants identified behaviors they thought the professionals used as criteria for assessing readiness for discharge. They then initiated these behaviors with the intention of convincing professionals of their readiness for discharge. The informants who exhibited taking charge behaviors were also those informants who described intrusive experiences.

The first of these informants felt that the professionals' criteria for his readiness to be discharged was his demonstrated ability to control his anger: "I think it was anger control—is the main thing that they are concerned about." His anger was associated with the threatening and punitive intrusive experiences which he attributed to others in his immediate environment. Although this informant did not think his reaction to these intrusions was inappropriate, he described purposefully controlling this reaction in order to prove his readiness to be discharged:

> In my case, I have to play a kitten and take shit and abuse from everybody. . . . In my case, that's like taking away the wings off an airplane. . . . In the—in the fact that I don't use it for aggression, I use it for self-defense.

> I was quiet and kept to myself—didn't lash out in anger at anybody. At least when I did, I made peace afterwards, which is exactly what I did today. He still thinks he's got one up on me, but I'm laughing inside at him anyway. It's a children's game.

The second informant believed that his attending physician wanted his "voices stopped" prior to his discharge: "They wanted to get those stopped." He initiated behaviors to convince his physician this had occurred:

> By just talking to him patiently and, um, telling him that, um, I wasn't hearing voices anymore. So I . . . told a little white lie, but I don't . . . need to be in hospital any longer. . . . Well . . . I just told them that just because they're asking me about my voices and, you know, I . . . don't hear them all the time anymore, you know. Um . . . just once in awhile I hear them, and they don't preoccupy me, so there's no problem there, you know.

Although the behaviors described by these informants were different, the intended effect was the same, that is, to convince the professionals of their readiness to be discharged.

Both of these informants avoided situations in which they would have to address the source of their psychological experiences:

> And she [physician] wouldn't believe me that there's a transmitter in my room, so I just refused to talk to her after awhile, you know.

When the second informant was told by professionals he was hallucinating, he said, "I just kept my mouth shut and grin and bear it." Following the physicians' authorization for their discharge, both of these informants said their attending physicians were on their side:

> I feel great now that Dr. _____ has realized I'm no longer a danger to myself or society. So she's on my side now.

> He's [physician] . . . basically looked at it in my . . . eyes and seen that I'm ready to go, so . . . I think he's carrying through with it, eh?

The fourth cell in figure 4.2 (Cell *d*) consists of patients who do not assess themselves as ready for discharge and do not consider it likely that they will be discharged. They were considered too sick, and they were excluded from the study. Ideally, during the course of recovery, patients move from Cell *d* to Cell *a* prior to leaving the hospital; however, the informants in this study moved from Cell *a* to Cell *c* when disagreements emerged between them and the hospital professionals regarding their readiness to leave the hospital. These disagreements were precipitated by rejection of candidacy for placement in alternative living accommodations.

To the informants in this study, being in the hospital was comparable to being in an army boot camp. In addition to organizational and structural similarities the primary function of both institutions is to prepare its service recipients for roles autonomous from institutional roles. The informants in this study sought discharge from the hospital when they assessed themselves ready to return to the community or when they felt their hospital treatment was not helping them return to the community. When the informants wished to attain a discharge from the hospital they displayed three types of getting out behaviors: marking time, breaking out, and taking charge.

Conclusion

All of the informants recalled pleasant experiences from their extended past. Moreover, they described this past as discontinuous from their preadmission past, which began with their first contact with formal mental health care. The preadmission past is an extended period of *not making it* in the community, culminating with their present admissions.

The actual and anticipated life experiences of the informants are schematically presented in Figure 4.3. The first row of circles (Figure 4.3) represents the life experiences of the informants who assessed themselves ready to return to the community. These informants were *anticipating mastery* of their community environments and characterized their immediate future as "new beginnings." Their life experiences, therefore, can be depicted as progressing linearly.

The second set of circles (Figure 4.3) represents the life experiences of the informant who did not assess himself ready to return to the community. This informant characterized his immediate future as a continuation of the preadmission "struggle to make it," and he predicted the need for future hospitalizations. Because he anticipated eventual acquisition of productive community roles, the circle representing his anticipated future is not obliterated by circles representing present hospital and preadmission experiences.

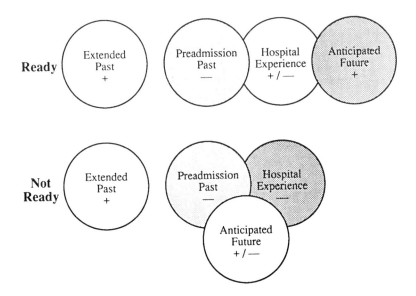

Figure 4.3. Actual and Anticipated Life Experiences of Informants

Becoming Ordinary

The core explanatory variable of the results was *becoming ordinary*. A process labeled *becoming ordinary* outwardly appeared to be paradoxical. Adults are not generally viewed as striving for ordinariness; rather, adults usually move toward outstanding life careers. When viewed from the informants' frame of reference, however, this concept lost much of its paradoxical impact. The informants' frame of reference was their preadmission experiences and all of them described themselves as failures during this extended time period because they were *not making it* in the community. Their admission to a hospital removed them from overwhelming community environments.

At predischarge all of the informants aspired to become self-supporting and independent; however, they did not all anticipate immediate progress toward *becoming ordinary*. The predischarge informants who were *anticipating mastery* of their communities were also anticipating immediate acquisition of productive commu-

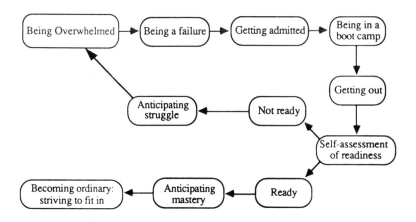

Figure 4.4. Flow Chart Depicting the Process of "Becoming Ordinary"

nity roles. From their perspective, they were *becoming ordinary.* The informant who was anticipating continuation of his preadmission struggle to *make it* in the community was not anticipating immediate progress toward *becoming ordinary.* Self-assessment of unreadiness to return to the community was accompanied by anticipated inability to manage in the community and the prediction of the need for future hospitalizations. Figure 4.4 schematically represents the process of *becoming ordinary.*

The concept *becoming ordinary* embodied the informants' perceptions of their anticipated future as well as their past experience and subsequently it was superordinate to all other concepts. To recapitulate, informants who characterized themselves as past failures in the community were anticipating assuming *ordinary* roles in the community. The informants in this study felt that *becoming ordinary* meant becoming normal, productive community members.

Note

1. The sample consisted of four males in their twenties and thirties, three of whom had been diagnosed with paranoid schizophrenia (the fourth participant was diagnosed with residual schizophrenia). All of the informants had lengthy histories of mental illness ranging from 3 to 15 years, were hospitalized at the time of the study,

and were awaiting discharge. Only one of the informants had admitted himself to the psychiatric care facility voluntarily. Each informant was interviewed a total of four to six times. Individuals with schizophrenia typically display less complex ideas, exhibit frequent speech errors, and tend to repeat themselves. For these reasons, the interview techniques typically used by grounded theorists were modified by the researcher to include frequent verbal probing and direct leading questions. All of the probes and direct questions, however, were grounded in previously obtained data.

References

Bland, R. C. (1984). Long term mental illness in Canada: An epidemiological perspective on schizophrenia and affective disorders. *Canadian Journal of Psychiatry, 29,* 242-246.

Bland, R. C., Parker, J. H., & Orn, H. (1976). Prognosis in schizophrenia: A ten-year follow-up of first admissions. *Archives of General Psychiatry, 33,* 949-954.

Bland, R. C., Parker, J. H., & Orn, H. (1978). Prognosis in schizophrenia: Prognostic predictors and outcome. *Archives of General Psychiatry, 35,* 72-77.

Cottman, S. B., & Mezey, A. G. (1976). Community care and the prognosis of schizophrenia. *Acta Psychiatrica Scandinavica, 53,* 95-104.

Green, R. S. (1984). Why schizophrenic patients should be told their diagnosis. *Hospital and Community Psychiatry, 35*(1), 76-77.

5

Mothers' Involvement in Their Adolescent Daughters' Abortions

JUDY NORRIS

Where do research questions come from? Ideally, they arise from observations in the clinical setting. In the case of this study, Norris observed mothers waiting for their daughters to return from the operating room where they had gone for a therapeutic abortion. The lack of support for these women, either from professionals or from friends and/or family members, was striking because the mothers appeared to be more distressed than their daughters. Wondering about how she could best help these women, Norris searched for material in the library and to her amazement found very little. It is these gaps in the literature that indicate the dire need for qualitative research.

The timing of in-depth, interactive interviews raises many ethical questions. In this study, Norris did not consider her role to be that of a counselor and she felt she should not be involved in the abortion decision-making process; therefore, her first contact with the mothers was after the procedure had commenced and her interviews were conducted by telephone one week later. During the interviews, however, she found it was easy to obtain retrospective accounts of the decision-making process as the mothers needed to tell their stories and consequently they began their stories at the beginning.

Although it was not Norris' intention, the process of telling the story was therapeutic for these women. Mothers began their stories tentatively but as they relaxed the words poured forth rapidly. As accounts progressed the

AUTHOR'S NOTE: Derived from: Norris, J. R. (1986). *The experience of mothers consenting for daughters' abortions*. Unpublished master's thesis, University of Alberta, Edmonton, Alberta, Canada.

This research was supported in part by the Alberta Foundation for Nursing Research.

*informants seemed to experience a release of pent-up emotions. All
interviews seemed to end on a light note, for example with humorous
banter about "why mothers of adolescent daughters go gray." Once or
twice, when Norris attempted a second interview, she discovered that the
mothers were not interested in talking about their experiences a second
time. It was as if there had been a grand catharsis in the first interview,
and having told the story the informants considered the issue closed.
Many of these women had not had the opportunity to tell their stories to
a compassionate listener. Some husbands, if told about the abortion,
were not a source of support because they considered abortion to be
a woman's matter for their wife "to take care of" and mothers were
often reluctant to confide in their relatives and friends. For these
reasons telephone counseling services would provide women with
the opportunity to talk out the abortion experiences anonymously
with a neutral listener.*

An unwed adolescent's pregnancy is a crisis that may affect the
family, particularly her mother. A mother may view a daughter's
adolescent pregnancy as a sign of her own inadequacy as a parent;
therefore, she is often ready to accept some of the blame for the
situation (Bryan-Logan & Dancy, 1974). Although the mother is
almost always the parent who participates in and implements an
abortion decision for adolescent minors (Rosen, 1980; Rosen, Benson, & Stack, 1982), only passing reference is made to parents in
studies of adolescent pregnancy resolution. Indeed, as adolescent
girls may require the consent of a parent or guardian for therapeutic
abortions,[1] it can be argued that the resolution of adolescent pregnancy is often a dyadic experience that has the potential to disrupt
the lives of both the mother and the daughter. Although numerous
investigations have focused on the needs and perceptions of adolescent girls who are pregnant, to date the dyadic nature of the abortion
experience for adolescent minors has been largely ignored. In order
to broaden our understanding of these dyads a qualitative study was
undertaken to explore the experiences of mothers who consent for
their daughters' abortions.[2]

Events Prior to the Pregnancy:
Suspecting Pregnancy

When the informants in this study were asked to tell their story almost all the mothers began with background information pertaining to their daughters' sexual activity and contraceptive efforts. Also, most of the mothers described the supportive-educative role they had assumed in pregnancy prevention and the observations that led them to suspect their daughters' pregnancies.

Assessing Sexual Activity and Contraceptive Effort

The mothers in this study were sensitive to indicators that their daughters were sexually active and they sought information about this as well as their daughters' contraceptive efforts:

> Well, what made us think about it was that she had a hickey on her neck, and I'd noticed this when we were in [city] at Christmas time. So then, I thought, "Gee, you know, we'd better sit down and talk. This looks like it's getting heavy." So when we got home, we discussed it, and we point blankly asked her if she was having sexual relations, and she admitted it; and so then, we asked her what she was doing to prevent pregnancy.

> I think that I was quite aware of the fact that she was sleeping with him when it happened, and I talked to her about it. . . . She assured me that she was using some means of birth control, but she didn't want to talk about it in very much detail. It was [an] "Oh, mother, I know what I'm doing" sort of reaction.

Being Open in Talking About Sexual Topics

Most of the informants said they had openly discussed sexual topics with their daughters and had assumed a supportive-educative role in pregnancy prevention. Some of the informants were frustrated in their attempts to discuss sexual topics because their daughters often resisted such discussions; and when they would discuss sexual topics, the daughters either did not absorb the information or they did not apply it:

I said, "Well, [daughter], we're going to talk this out even though it is embarrassing for you. . . . I've got things that I want to say." And she'd say, "Yeah, yeah, yeah," and she'd let me go ahead and say these things [about birth control], but it's an "I know better" attitude. And they don't. . . . They are not nearly as well educated as they think. I was really surprised.

I have a fairly up-to-date attitude about premarital sex. We were just surprised to find out how poorly educated she actually was about the whole thing, and that surprised me . . . after all the talks we've had. . . . It really surprised me. Can you tie them to a chair and make them listen?

You know, it is so amazing that you can give the information, and in fact, in my case, I insisted that the information be there, and yet it [pregnancy] happened.

Only one daughter approached her mother to discuss contraceptives:

She said, "Mom, I've been going out with him for six months, and sometimes things get a bit tense, and I think I should go to the doctor and get the pill or something because I don't want to take a chance." And I said, "Fine . . . that's the attitude you should have, go talk to Dr. ____."

Some of the informants felt regret because they had not addressed the contraceptive issue early enough, because they had not been more assertive, or because they had accepted false indicators that suggested pregnancy would not occur:

I felt really badly that I hadn't talked to her about the pill, which I had promised myself over the years that I would do it if I had a daughter. . . . But you don't realize how fast they grow up.

She said they were using a condom, but she didn't say "sometimes" to me. She said they'd been using it, so I said, well, everything was okay. You know . . . sort of hoping it was quite safe.

Some of the mothers in this study felt their daughters were too young for sexual activity, and as a result, they had trouble advocating contraception:

So many times I wanted to go into her room and say, "Can we talk? Can we talk about birth control?" But then I'd think, no, she's too young. And she wasn't. That's something I regret. But birth control. It's like saying I give you my blessing.

Too bad they're starting [sexual activity] too young. Like, this happened with our daughter. . . . We told her to talk to us . . . to come to us when she thought that maybe it was time to get on the pill, before things went any further with her boyfriend; but she also knew that we thought she was too young to get into any sexual activity.

Unfortunately the daughter in the second example was placed in an untenable position, in a double-bind situation.

Monitoring

Many of the mothers were sensitive to changes in their daughters, either of an emotional or physical nature. They noticed the absence of menstruation and they suspected pregnancy when their daughters displayed symptoms such as vomiting, tiredness, or changes in body shape:

So then, I noticed that there was no tampons missing, and I kept asking her, "Have you got your period yet?" And she said, "No." I bought a home pregnancy test downtown, and we had done that, and it showed negative, so I figured that maybe she's just "off." I was when I was very young. . . . I'd get them every three months when I was 13, 14, 15, and so since I wasn't very regular, I thought that she's the same thing, but what really seriously made me think that she may be pregnant was around the first part of February . . . I noticed that she wasn't interested in going out anymore. At night she was so tired that she was going to sleep before her time. And she complained that her bras weren't fitting her properly and were too tight . . . you know, some of the symptoms. So that's when I really started seriously thinking about it, and then nothing was coming as far as the periods, [so] she saw the doctor.

I've kept this to myself, but being a mother who washes her daughters' clothes, I do know when they have their monthlies. And I noticed that [daughter] didn't have anything on her clothes. I flashed through my mind [that she was pregnant]. . . . I certainly didn't want to believe it.

The mothers in this study said they had taken some responsibility for preventing their daughters' pregnancies by employing two strategies: informing and being vigilant.

Informing

Although the results of several studies (Bloch, 1972; Herold, 1981; Herold & Goodwin, 1980) indicate that adolescents felt their mothers had been a poor source of information about sexual topics and contraception, most of the mothers in this study said their daughters resisted discussions about sex and frustrated their attempts to impart information about sexual topics. Some of the informants regretted having backed down when their daughters became embarrassed, protested that their privacy was being invaded, or stated that they "knew what they were doing."

Some investigators (Herold, 1984; Marsman, 1983; Reiss, 1973) have suggested that adolescents keep information about their sexual and contraceptive activities hidden from parents because they believe their parents would disapprove of their having intercourse. In this study two of the mothers explicitly stated their ambivalence about condoning contraception as they felt their daughters were too young to be sexually active. Also, several of the mothers in this study had offered to supply their daughters with information about contraceptive methods while at the same time directly or indirectly communicating their disapproval of premarital sexual activity. As a result, these daughters were put in an untenable position. As Lindemann (1974) says:

> A girl cannot readily ask her parents about birth control. They are usually ambivalent about, if not downright opposed to premarital sex. Even in families that have a permissive attitude toward premarital sex, parents are not able to help their daughters plan for birth control in concrete terms. (p. 29)

In this study only one daughter reportedly approached her mother to obtain contraceptive advice. In the other families in this study in which this issue was discussed, it was the *mother* who actively sought evidence of her daughter's sexual activity and contraceptive efforts and then attempted to inform her daughter about contraceptives and, in some cases, to assist her in obtaining them. Most of the mothers in this study, aware that their adolescent daughters would be unlikely to make such a revelation, took responsibility for assessing the situation and for intervening in order to prevent pregnancy regardless of their attitudes toward their daughters' premarital sexual activity. Pregnancy prevention was the salient concern.

It has been suggested that some mothers adopt an "ostrich response" to their daughters sexual behavior; that is, they protect themselves from knowledge about their daughters' sexual behavior while passively hoping they do not become pregnant (Bernard, 1975). In this study this phenomenon was demonstrated by a small minority of mothers who stated that they had never thought of their daughters as being sexually active and had, therefore, not discussed contraception with them in a situation-specific way. Although Herold and Way (1983) suggest that daughters discuss premarital sex and contraception with their mothers on a general level, with the personal details of the daughters' sexual behavior omitted, this was not the case in this present study: Those mothers who discussed premarital sex and contraception with their daughters applied their teaching specifically to the daughters' sexual behavior. Only those informants who were unaware of their daughters' sexual activity discussed these matters in general terms.

All the daughters in this study became pregnant as the result of unprotected intercourse. Parental variables such as perceived support of an adolescent female's decision to use a contraceptive method (Jorgensen & Sonstegard, 1984) and accompanying the adolescent to the birth control clinic (Scher, Emans, & Grace, 1984) were found to be predictors of more consistent contraceptive behavior in adolescents. Although many of the mothers had supported the use of contraception, only one mother in this study said that she had accompanied her daughter to the family physician specifically to obtain contraceptives. Two informants told their family physicians that their daughters had permission to obtain contraceptives, although the other mothers who discussed this topic delegated the responsibility for obtaining contraceptives to the daughter.

The informants were astonished that their daughters became pregnant from unprotected intercourse after they had informed them about contraceptives and advocated their use. Their daughters' actions, however, reveal the adolescents' difficulty with using contraceptives.

In this study one daughter used condoms sometimes, one was taking the birth control pill irregularly, three had prescriptions for the pill but had quit taking it, and the other eight were not using contraceptives. Youngs and Niebyl (1975) note that a common clinical problem is the adolescent who presents with an unwanted pregnancy as the result of an irregular use of the birth control pill.

Being Vigilant

Fox (1980) describes the conflict of two aspects of the mother role in a daughter's transition from child to adult, a conflict that involves deciding whether to act as protector of daughter-as-child making decisions on her behalf, or to act as guide to the daughter-as-woman allowing her to find her own way and live with the consequences of her decisions. The informants in this study maneuvered along this fine line using the strategy of *being vigilant*. In the role of protector the informants attempted to teach their daughters the norms, values, and expectations of the family culture in order to avoid an unwanted adolescent pregnancy. This was done by discussing sexual topics, contraception, and the consequences of adolescent pregnancy. In the role of guide toward competence in the adult sexual role, the mothers in this study sought indicators that their daughters were assuming responsibility for their sexual behavior so that they could delegate responsibility accordingly. The mothers overtly assessed their daughters' competence in sexual matters by inquiring about their daughters' sexual activity and their knowledge and use of contraceptive methods and they covertly assessed their daughters' competency by *being vigilant*. The informants in this study knew when their daughters' menstruation should occur, were sensitive to indicators that they were sexually active, and attempted to monitor their boyfriends, friends, and life-styles.

Eight of the informants said they had suspected that their daughters were pregnant when they noticed the absence of menstruation and saw symptoms such as vomiting, tiredness, or changes in body shape. All of the mothers who suspected pregnancy took action to confirm their suspicions, either by taking their daughters to physicians or by using drugstore pregnancy tests.

Many of the daughters in this study were described by their mothers as talented girls who were doing well in school and had plans for postsecondary education. Therefore, *being vigilant* was a protective device used by the informants in this study; and by using this strategy these mothers allowed their daughters to develop autonomy and separation while keeping a maternal safety net under them. In other words, the main objective of the mothers in this study was to prevent pregnancy from interfering with their daughters' life options.

The Pregnancy: Taking Responsibility

Finding Out

The fact that they had suspected their daughters were pregnant did not prevent the mothers in this study from reacting with strong emotions when the pregnancy was finally confirmed. Some mothers reported being shocked, devastated, or angry, although others experienced shock reactions later:

> I was devastated when I first heard it, even though I was possibly expecting it. I was hoping to walk into the doctor's office and hear that it wasn't true . . . but it was, so I was . . . like I couldn't say anything. I was so speechless at first.

Pregnancy Resolution Decision Making

Considering the Alternatives

When considering the alternatives the mothers in this study said they, their daughter, and others in the family examined the context of the pregnancy, that is how the resolution decision would ultimately affect others including the fetus. Three alternatives were available and discussed by these families: pregnancy continuation with the child being relinquished for adoption, pregnancy continuation with the child being kept, and abortion.

Pregnancy Continuation with Adoption

Adoption was not considered by any of the families; in each family, either the mother, the daughter, or the father was against this alternative. In each case the fetus was considered as a potential family member who should not be separated from its kin:

We didn't even discuss adoption because it would have never happened. . . . We'd have probably gone through the whole role, the interviews, whatever, about being adopted, but when the time came, the baby wouldn't have been adopted because my husband would have said, "That's our grandchild . . . it can come home with us . . . it won't go to another home." So we didn't even discuss it.

Well, I just couldn't let . . . her go through the pregnancy and carry the child that long and then have given it up, and her not seeing it, and probably me not seeing it and knowing that there's a child out somewhere. . . . I know that whoever adopted it would love it and take care of it, but still, I felt that there is something out there that belongs to me, to us, to her, and I'd not be able to see it.

One family considered the alternative of pregnancy continuation with adoption for financial reasons, but this option was abandoned when the daughter, herself an adoptee, objected:

Her dad was with me, of course, and we're all sitting there, and her dad suggested, "Well, you can go through the pregnancy, but we cannot afford to keep the baby." . . . She [daughter] said, "You know, if I go through this, it is going to be so hard to give it up."

Pregnancy Continuation with the Child being Kept

The mothers in this study said that pregnancy continuation with the child being kept was considered a poor alternative for several reasons, the main one being the adverse effect on their daughters' life options. Most of the informants felt that their daughters were not mature enough to provide good mothering for a child and some mothers were against taking on infant care at their stage in life:

I hoped that she would make the decision she made. I didn't want to lead her, but I hoped that she would make that decision because although I have a tremendous respect for life, I also felt that at the age of seventeen she wouldn't be able to provide any kind of a decent life for a youngster nor would it do her any good to have her life changed as drastically as having a baby of her own would.

I would say that no that would not be an acceptable solution [for mother to take on care of baby], but then, I wouldn't know unless I was put in it.

I mean, some things you have to accept whether you want to or not, but I would not have been prepared to raise a child at my stage in life. That really wouldn't have been acceptable.

One informant mentioned marriage as a solution to the problem, but she said that both she and her husband had emphatically rejected the idea:

And the only thing my husband and I completely agreed on was that certainly no marriage at that age. That was something we were both adamant about.

Abortion

Ultimately, all the families in this study chose abortions as the best pregnancy resolution decision; however, there was considerable variation in the amount of deliberation required and the degree of consensus within the family:

I felt she had made a mistake, and she was going about it the best way to correct it, and so I was relieved that she was going that way.

I did not want the baby knowing who the father was. I did not want any part of that baby, you know. Like I told her, "I'll hate it." Maybe . . . that is the first thing I thought of when she told me: "She's having an abortion." . . . When I found out who it was, you know, and not only for the reason of that, but I could *not* see her going through a pregnancy. I just couldn't see it. It was just *impossible*. Not *her,* you know? And she's got so much going for her that all I could think of is that it is going to ruin her life.

You just hope it was the right one [decision], and in our case, I'm sure it was because I haven't been working except for part-time for the last two and a half years, and money-wise we just do not have what it takes to even do the necessities for a child.

Mothers' Involvement in the Resolution Decision

There was considerable variation in the extent to which mothers had input into the choice of abortion as the pregnancy resolution decision. Three informants said their daughters had chosen abortion with no alternatives being discussed by the family. These mothers were, therefore, not involved in the decision:

> No, she didn't say she wanted an abortion, she said she was *going* to have an abortion. So we were told, not consulted at all, but I can't remember the gist of the conversation, but we agreed that we would pursue that.

> She left us no choice in the matter. She told us right out what she wanted and that was that. We talked and talked to her and tried to change her mind, but there was no way.

In three families, although the daughter chose abortion alternatives were discussed:

> She had [written] down that she had made her decision. She had expressed that . . . she was only seventeen years old, and if [she] wanted to get a decent job, [she] would have to continue school, and who would be left looking after the baby . . . me and this boy's parents. But she didn't feel it was right to burden . . . us because she knew that me and my husband were enjoying ourselves. You know, we'd gone on trips, and we could go out in the evenings and didn't have to worry. So then we just discussed it, and she said she didn't want to have the baby, and I wasn't for abortion. And then I talked to the doctor, and he felt being that she was at that age that it was best. And then we just went ahead with it.

One informant made the decision that her daughter would have an abortion. Eventually, the daughter agreed with this choice:

> She didn't know which way to go, you know. Should she go with it, or should she have the abortion? But I guess what really helped her make up her mind was that after we talked to the doctor, I think she knew that I didn't want her to go through with the pregnancy, and she went my way, and mind you, now she says, "I couldn't have gone through it. I want to finish school, and I don't want to leave that school that I'm at." She'd of had to leave that school, and she wants to go through school and get a good job, you know. She didn't want to be a drop-out. I felt like maybe I'm really being nasty, dirty, doing this to her, you know, making her have the abortion . . . well, not making her, but making her decide. . . . "Okay, [daughter], you're going to make this decision because I don't want you to go through this [pregnancy]."

Four informants advocated abortion but they insisted that it be their daughters' decision:

> Well, I thought it was an awfully big decision for her to be making. I guess I probably felt sorry for her. I hoped that she would make the decision she made. I didn't want to lead her, but I hoped that she would make that decision [to abort].

> And then she went to the doctor and found out, and I asked her what . . . her decision was, what she was going to do, and she said that she wanted to have the abortion. So it was her decision, but possibly I prompted her in that direction. She may have thought that I would disapprove.

One informant and her daughter made the decision together after considering all alternatives:

> She asked me what I thought was the best thing to do, and I told her that's what I thought [advocated abortion], and I figured out for myself what's the best for her at her age, and this is the decision that we did make. Both of us, between the two of us. She didn't pressure me into it too much. . . . I mean, she told me what she wanted to do, what she would like to do, [but] she didn't press me into it.

One informant said the pregnancy resolution decision was made by the whole family: "[The] whole family was involved, and we just decided that it was best that she had an abortion."

The Man Involved in the Pregnancy

Most of the mothers in this study were angry at the man involved in the pregnancy. He was often viewed as a predatory male who had taken advantage of their daughter. Most of the informants despised him and hoped their daughter would not see him again. None of the families considered him when making the pregnancy resolution decision. He was an outsider:

> My main concern now is that she'll get an ounce of intelligence in her and realize that he's just a bum.

I know it's over with, but I am angry with him. . . . I still am, and he has to do a lot to earn any respect from me, and until he earns that, I really never want to see him. The thing is he's not mean, he's not nasty, he is actually a kind person, but he's a *bum,* that's all. Maybe I can explain that: He's not dirty, he's a very clean person, but if he doesn't have to work, or as long as someone will feed him and entertain him and whatever, he's quite happy to live that way. I don't need a son-in-law like that. . . . I know my daughter has learned a lesson, and I think and I'm hoping in a month he won't even exist in her mind.

Three mothers said they were so angry with the man involved in the pregnancy that they wanted to physically attack him:

You know, to this day, if I ever see him, I think I'll have to go beat him up. I mean, he's six feet tall, and I'm only five feet tall, but I am still going to beat him up and say, *"Why did you hurt her?"*

I keep threatening my daughters . . . every once in a while . . . maybe I say it twice a day, maybe I don't say it one day, and maybe the next day it's five times a day, but I'm going to punch his teeth in. He better not cross my path.

Two mothers were not angry with the man involved in the pregnancy, and these mothers saw the pregnancy as mutually caused or, in one case, as a mistake made by two very young adolescents:

Well, they just had their one year anniversary about a week ago. . . . It wasn't a casual thing, she's been with him, and it didn't break it up. He offered to go to the hospital with her. I don't know if she talked it over with him at all. It was my feeling that it was totally her decision.

The boy that was responsible . . . he knew, but his parents didn't, and we sort of set the foot down yesterday and told her to talk to him, and we thought his parents had the right to know what happened as well, and so he finally talked to his mother last night, and I guess she was happy to hear about it, you know, that she was told, but she seems to think as well that the right thing was done because of their ages. The boy is only sixteen.

Daughter's Father or the Man in Mother's Life

The daughter's father or the man in the mother's life was considered a very influential part of the situation by the informants in this study. These men were described as strongly stating and sometimes enforcing their views about the daughters' pregnancies and resolution decisions. Some of the mothers in this study said they agreed to the abortion decision only because the man was adamant that the pregnancy be resolved in this way. None of the daughters told the man about her pregnancy; in families where he was informed the mother disclosed this information:

> I told her that we had to talk with dad . . . which she was afraid of. . . . I don't know why, but she was afraid to tell her dad, but then at first she was afraid to tell me as well.

> Well, I'm the one who told him. We were alone at the time, and I told him, and I thought for sure he was going to cry he was so hurt. When I did tell it to him, he was sitting on the couch, and he jumped right up, and he grabbed his chest, and that kind of scared me. . . . I thought, "Oh my God, no." But right away, he asked who it was, and that made him madder yet.

In three of the families the man was not informed of the pregnancy, each for a different reason: mother and daughter both felt that the father would "kick the daughter out of the house," the mother and daughter were living apart from the father and felt it was inadvisable to inform him, the daughter's father was dead and the mother felt that their daughter's pregnancy would adversely affect the man's [mother's primary relationship] attitude toward the daughter:

> We wouldn't have done this except that her dad was so against it, you know, and would have kicked her right out of the house.

> Well, this is the first time I've had to keep something back from him . . . the very first time. It's not that . . . I would love to tell him and be honest about it, but I don't think it's fair to [daughter] to tell him because I don't want an added pressure between them.

Fathers' Input Into Pregnancy Resolution Decision

The mothers in this study said that all the men (except two) who knew of the pregnancies advocated abortion: one man thought the daughter should have the baby to "teach her a lesson" and another suggested pregnancy continuation with the baby being relinquished for adoption. According to the informants, these men also considered the consequences of the pregnancy to all concerned including the fetus:

> We talked about it again for the afternoon when him and I were alone, and he said, "Yeah, it would be kinda nice, you know, to have a grandchild," but . . . he thinks that it's best for her. . . . She's only fourteen years old.

> He [husband] thinks more ahead and what it's going to do in the future to the whole family, actually, 'cause she's still got three and a half years of school, plus a couple years of college, so we could have figured on looking after the baby for at least five years.

When discussing the extent of the man's input into the pregnancy resolution decision two mothers said that if their daughters had continued the pregnancy and kept the child then their own primary relationship might have been threatened:

> You are the first one I'm saying it to [and that is] that if she had decided to keep this baby what would have happened between [man who is mother's primary relationship] and myself in our relationship? Really, I honestly do *not* know. As strong a relationship as this is, it has been seven years we've been seeing one another, what kind of pressure it would have put on? Would we have been able to see it through? I *don't* know.

> And being my husband felt so much the other way [that daughter should have abortion], I don't know. It might have caused trouble with us [if daughter kept baby]. I don't know.

Mothers Supporting Daughters

Although some of the daughters in this study were close to eighteen years of age, most of the informants referred to their daughters as "babies," "children," "youngsters," or "little girls." Perceiving that their daughters were not equipped to resolve the crisis of an unwanted pregnancy unaided, the mothers accepted the problem as their own, taking responsibility for the situation:

> I guess [I took responsibility] because I still feel that at seventeen she is still too immature to fully accept the fact of what she is doing, and I still

feel that I'm the one that is still making a lot of decisions for her. And I think I'll probably feel that way for a long time.

I just don't want them [daughters] to be hurt, and if I accept this responsibility, then they're going to be all right. I can handle it, and they can't. That's the way I feel. If I take the responsibility, then she can go on and enjoy the best years of her life, and I can cope with it.

Besides sharing their daughters' crisis of an unwanted adolescent pregnancy and assisting them with the complicated arrangements necessary for a therapeutic abortion, the mothers in this study were sensitive caregivers concerned with their daughters' physical and emotional well-being. They comforted their daughters by giving emotional support and by providing physical nearness:

And when she came home from school, she just walked into her room. So we both went in and told her that we did love her and would stand by her, and we thought she made the right decision to terminate the pregnancy.

Finally, one day . . . we were alone, and she [told] me that she was pregnant, and we were sitting side by side, and I grabbed her, and I hugged her, and I told her, "Look, just because this happened, you know, we're going to love you just as much as before."

The night that she came home from the hospital she was in my room, and my husband surprisingly said to me, "You should sleep with [daughter] tonight." So I went in, and I got into bed, and I thought, "I'm not going to press it if she doesn't want me here," but surprisingly, she did. You know, we haven't slept in the same bed in years. . . . Since she was a little baby.

The Abortion: Consenting

All of the mothers in this study were facing the reality of abortion for the first time. Although many of the mothers in the study said that their daughters knew girls who had had abortions, most of the informants had not been involved with an abortion, either through relatives or friends. As a personal experience abortion was foreign to the informants; it was an event they had never expected to encounter:

It happens to other people, like car accidents. I didn't think I would ever have to be confronted with anything like this, but a lot I knew.

I found it very interesting [television program about abortion], and I wanted to see the pros and cons of abortion, never thinking that within six months I'd be going through this with my daughter.

The Mothers' Views on Abortion

All but three mothers expressed their personal opposition to abortion; nonetheless, they all felt that it was the best pregnancy resolution choice for their daughters. Three mothers had "pro-choice" views and they said that they had no problem with the decision to abort. One mother, who had espoused a pro-choice view prior to her daughter's pregnancy, reversed her stance when confronted with the reality of abortion:

I think it was the right thing to do, although I'm against abortion.

At first, you know, I wasn't willing to go to that part . . . for her to have this done. Because, actually, to tell the truth, I don't believe in it [abortion], I never did. So it was quite a decision to have to make on my part.

I think my attitude about abortion has always been what it is right now. I don't think I ever really struggled. If a person is pregnant and wants to do something about it, I think that that right is theirs. . . . I have a fairly strong religious belief and background, and that has never entered into it. I've always felt very, very strongly that it is the woman's decision to make. It's her body. She's the one that has to care for the child after it is born. She has to decide if she's capable of going through with this whole thing, and I think I've got a simplistic attitude toward it, but very simply, that's what it is, and I don't have a whole lot of hang-ups about it, and probably, I've passed this on to my kids.

I think I've changed my attitude over abortion. I've watched shows lately on abortions, and I've always just had the attitude that it's a woman's body and she can do what she wants with it. . . . But I've never had to face it before.

Secrecy

Secrecy about the pregnancy and abortion concerned all the informants and their daughters in this study. Some made elaborate plans to keep the pregnancy and the abortion secret; for example, even when some of the daughters felt ill they continued to go to school. In the interest of maintaining secrecy some of the mothers did not seek support for themselves; one mother did not stay at the hospital during the abortion procedure so that the neighbors would see no difference in her normal routine:

> No, I didn't want to discuss it with anyone. This town is only about 6,000 people, and in fact, I wouldn't be surprised if it got around anyway because of the clinic itself. You know, people that work there.

> There was no way I could discuss *this* with her [a relative] because most people will condemn you and don't really put themselves in that position of what they would do.

> I was sorry that I couldn't stay with her the whole time, but we're trying to not let anybody know, and you know, we wanted to carry on as normal as possible.

Support for the Mothers

An important issue was the conflict between the desire to keep the abortion a secret and the need to talk to someone:

> She didn't want anybody else to know about it. We respected that. Although it doesn't give me . . . someone to talk to about it.

> We did keep it very much to ourselves, and *that* was the hard part.

> And she [daughter] asked me not to tell anybody, and I said at the moment that I would agree not to tell anybody because I didn't know what to . . . and I realized the next day that I was in shock about the whole thing, and I realized that I . . . literally did not know which way to turn, and I needed to talk to somebody, but I thought that I needed to respect my promise to her.

Some of the women in this study said their husbands had been a source of support; however, some informants felt that they had to support both their daughter and their husband as well as deal with their own feelings:

We [mother and her husband] thought it was something we should do together. As far as going through this, it was done together.

When we first found out she was pregnant, she said, "Do we have to tell anybody?" And I said, "Yes, I have to tell your dad because this is something I feel I can't go through alone. I'm going to need some support."

He was supportive in that it was sort of "I know what you're going through, hon, and I know that this is tough, and gee, what's for dinner?" He's that kind of a person, anyway, though. I knew that I'd get somebody that I could lean on to a certain degree.

Some of the informants felt that the men in their lives would not be a satisfactory source of support in this situation. These women wished they could have talked to a woman about their feelings, especially a woman who had borne children or had gone through the same experience:

But I think what I thought when they took [daughter] in for the surgery, I think that's when I could have talked to somebody. Really, really talked to somebody. My husband was there, but I just couldn't tell him what was in my mind. I think only a woman who has children and has had them, you know, I don't think he could understand for a man.

I think I would have liked to talk to someone who had been through it that could have assured me that . . . not that I was doing the right thing, but that "yeah, this too shall pass, and you will feel . . . life will be normal again and what you're feeling right now *is* okay and it *is* normal. It's okay to feel frustrated and sad about it." And my God, how could this have happened? Where did I let her down? Where did I go wrong? What didn't I do as a mother? All those questions were *really* difficult to deal with, and I realized after it was over that this wasn't an issue that I had to take up with myself, it was something that had happened that had to be dealt with, it was simple as that. I was questioning very, very, very much where had I let this kid down? Where had I been a really poor mother? And *that* would have been helpful . . . to have somebody say, "Whoa, your thinking is a little screwed up here."

Two mothers said that they had felt no need for support for themselves; however, both these women had previously reported extensive family support:

I don't know that I felt the need for support. I think she felt the need for support, and maybe because I was supporting her, I didn't feel it myself.

No, I didn't [feel a need for support] because like I said we're very, very close, and we shared it. We went through it all together, and I guess I was lucky that way.

Consenting for Daughters' Abortions

Because their daughters were under the age of eighteen and not emancipated, each mother in this study gave formal informed consent for her daughters to undergo the abortion procedure. The signing of the consent form implicated the mothers in a personal, concrete way, and their varied responses reflect their underlying feelings about abortion.

For some mothers the act of consenting meant that they were helping their daughters, and in this context none of the women were in conflict with the idea of abortion:

It [consenting] reinforced for me that I'm here because I want to be here. She is still my daughter and my little girl. I wouldn't want to be anywhere else but here, and I am taking responsibility for her and for her error.

I thought she was doing the right thing, so the right thing for me to do was to sign it. I didn't feel there was any reason I shouldn't, so I didn't feel bad in any way.

Those informants who said they believed abortion to be morally wrong felt that they were now morally compromised as the result of having given consent. One woman felt that all her moral beliefs had crumbled:

Abortion is very much against my religious beliefs for one thing, and so I feel that I have to live with something that I did very wrong.

I think that was the point [signing consent] at which I realized that I was doing it, and it was something that I was going to have to live with the rest of my life.

Other informants who had fewer problems with the idea of abortion than those who believed it to be morally wrong consented for their daughters' sake, even though this decision was against their own beliefs:

And so I thought it over, and I didn't want to sign for it because I'm against abortion, but I thought of her age, and she is still going to school, and it wasn't too long in the pregnancy, so I agreed to it, and that's how it came about.

I don't care for it [abortion], but this time . . . I was concerned with [daughter's] health. I'm sure that she would have been down and depressed because she didn't want this to happen, but it did, and . . . she wants to finish her schooling which she needs bad . . . nowadays. I felt that I was doin' the wrong thing, but for her sake, I done it because I know that in the end it is better for her this way.

One woman felt extremely relieved when signing the consent form because signing meant that the abortion was actually going to happen:

[When signing the consent] I felt 500,000 tons off my back, that it was finally happening, and that it was going to be over in a couple hours.

Waiting For the Abortion To Take Place

The mothers in this study said two waiting periods were stressful times for them. The first, waiting for the Therapeutic Abortion Committee's (TAC) approval, caused anxiety for several mothers and they experienced relief when approval for the abortion procedure was confirmed:

The waiting, the waiting. Was she going to be accepted or not?

It was . . . so hard, but like I said, it's the waiting period, wondering if she was accepted or not. That was the hard part.

I was worried, if she's turned down, what's my husband going to say?

The other waiting period, after the TAC's approval but before the abortion took place, was a stressful time for the two mothers who had reservations about the abortion decision:

Actually, I guess, I was hoping she would change her mind. That's what I was doing. Yeah. Kinda hoping my husband would phone up and say, no, he doesn't want to do it, and we won't. That was my reaction, so it was just sitting here waiting for it to happen, I guess.

The night before we were all a little jumpy. We were all very quiet. The way I felt was almost like someone was going to die.

The Day of the Abortion

Reactions at the Hospital

The Environment

Virtually all the mothers in this study were distressed by the admission procedure. They felt vulnerable in the admissions waiting area, which they described as public, stark, impersonal, and crowded:

I felt somewhat like we were being herded around like cattle.

There is a lot of people there coming in in the morning, and you feel, well, are they here for the same reason? Do they know why she's here? People are all being admitted, you know? And you don't want anybody to know. And you are wondering, do they know?

One of the reasons I found it so tough, like I said, was walking in in the morning and seeing this line of young children, of babies, waiting to have abortions. It just about knocked my teeth out. In fact, I wondered . . . I said, "Oh, jeepers, this can't all be for the same reason," but I found out as the day went on that, yep, same reason. And from that point on, I really went into a little bit of shock.

Two mothers said that they became impatient waiting for their daughters' discharge from the hospital:

At one point I found myself getting annoyed because I wanted to go home, and I wanted her to start feeling better so we could get the hell out of there. I was getting to that point . . . I was really getting antsy to leave. I felt like I'd been there long enough. I'd done my duty, and I wanted to go.

The Staff

The mothers seemed to expect censure from the nursing staff and they were prepared to protect their daughters from any mistreatment that might occur. The reactions to the staff varied from descriptions of "wonderful" to criticisms of the nurses for having no compassion, not being motherly, or being "clinical." One mother had wished for more contact with the surgeon:

The nurses at the hospital . . . were so understanding, they were so nice. . . . I was afraid of when she went in that day that they'd be nasty to her because I've heard some people say, "You know, that nurse, she was so mean to me because I had this done," and I went in there thinking don't you dare hurt her or anything, or I'm going to let you have it. I mean this little girl . . . it was an accident, more or less, and don't you dare do anything to her, but they were so nice.

I found that some of the nursing staff could have been, how can I put it, they could have had more compassion. Like, I seen a few girls there that . . . didn't [have] any parents with them, and . . . they [the nurses] could have had more compassion. Like, I realize that these girls are teenagers, they're teenyboppers, and they are having abortions, but well, they choose to work on that unit, and I believe they could show more compassion. And I also believe that after the surgery that the surgeon could come and speak to the patient or the parent or both. That didn't happen.

Fears and Worries

Many of the mothers in this study said they had been extremely worried about their daughters' safety in the operating room. One mother worried that her daughter would be frightened, and another mother was afraid her daughter might be unable to conceive again after the abortion:

I sort of had this fear that the wrath of God was going to come down on me, and maybe she won't come out alive.

I was really worried about her going for the abortion. I thought, what if something goes wrong? What if something goes wrong, and they come back and tell me she didn't make it? All these things go through your mind, you know.

There's always a chance that she can never have another one. That was one of my worries.

Mothers' Observations of Daughters

The mothers in this study sought indicators that their daughters appreciated the implications of the abortion. They looked for evidence that the daughter "knew what she had done" and was affected by it in some way, perhaps by feeling a loss:

I looked at my daughter, and I feel that she doesn't realize exactly what's happening, but I've had two children, I know what's happening.

When I came back to the room, the nurse had just finished cleaning her up, and she was sobbing. Just sobbing. I wanted to say, "What do you feel?" I wanted to know did she feel a sense of loss? Well, I would still like to ask this question to her, and I still haven't. . . . *Does* she feel a sense of loss? Being a normal mother, what came out of my mouth was "Are you in any pain?" And she said, "Yes," and I don't think she was. I think this because when we got home she didn't seem to have pain, and she said for supper she wanted Chinese food, so if she was in any discomfort whatsoever, she would never eat.

Some of the fathers were present with the mothers during their daughters' stay in the hospital. The informants said that the fathers were worried about their daughters' safety and they seemed to be emotionally upset:

He didn't realize that she had gone for the surgery. I didn't say, you know, I just sat there, and I started to cry. And when we were having coffee I told him, I said, "I hope the surgery is going all right," and . . . it was almost like he wanted to jump up and say "Stop!" That was the impression I got. He didn't say it, but after eighteen years you know. But then he just said, "I hope everything goes all right."

My husband said all he was worried about was her getting through the surgery without breathing problems. Since this happened, my husband has been doing a lot of drinking, a *lot*, every day, as a matter of fact, and I had said to him the other day, "I think we'd better have a talk," and the next day he didn't drink, and last night, only one beer. [Maybe] he knew I'd noticed the drinking, but maybe this is his way of coping. I know his mother was really, really against abortion, and he knew that because she had talked to him about it. Hopefully, someday he'll talk about it . . . he just takes a long time to sort out his feelings.

The Fetus

Almost all of the mothers openly considered the fetus. Some of the informants said they did not allow themselves to think of it as a baby and that this was a protection device. Other mothers said they they felt it best to deal directly with the issue of the fetus or those feelings might come out later and cause problems:

It's like part of me is gone . . . and she's my daughter, and I guess you'd consider it my grandchild.

I was just judging the moment they were coming for her, and something inside of me was screaming to stop *this,* but I knew I couldn't. I kept thinking this was my grandchild. This is murder. This is murder, you know. I never thought of that in those terms before. What I'm doing is murder. I just kept saying, "It's murder," and I still feel like I left somebody in that hospital, and I didn't want to.

There was a member of the family, and there is nothing you can do to bring him back.

I think . . . the more a person talks about it, so that they are not holding all those uncertain feelings inside, and that it does definitely help. You can have an abortion, but fifteen or ten years later, whatever, I think that in the back of your mind you will always remember and wonder.

Events After the Abortion:
Reconciling the Abortion

The period immediately following the abortion was a time of reorganization characterized by a desire for life to return to normal. This was expressed in a delightful way by one mother:

And the family is getting back. . . . It's like you took a jug and broke it, and now you're gluing it back together.

During this time the mothers in this study attempted to reconcile the abortion, dealt with their feelings about the event, and sought closure. Simultaneously, they reformulated strategies directed toward their daughters' pregnancy prevention. In other words, the informants felt this must *never* happen again.

Reconciling the Abortion

Grieving

The informants who said they were grieving related this emotion to the fetus. One mother, however, said that she had grieved for her daughter's "lost childhood":

I think you do have to grieve. I feel like it was me who had this done.

Maybe this two weeks of sitting around crying and burying my head under the pillow, maybe that was what I did need, maybe I needed that time to grieve. I couldn't stop myself. I'd jump up and say this is enough, and instead, I'd be sitting down crying again, so, yeah, I think you have to [grieve], I really, really do. It is like a death, a tragedy.

Well, I have grieved, and I'm sure I haven't stopped. I don't dwell on it, but I definitely grieved. I guess I would like to see her grieve a little. Well, she'll never be the same. It doesn't matter if you consider this . . . she's never going to be the same as what she was, and so her childhood is like ground unceremoniously to a halt.

Relief

The informants felt relief that the crisis of the unwanted pregnancy was resolved and that their daughters were going to be all right. But even though they thought the right decision had been made, they also thought this must never happen again; and most of the informants remained opposed to abortion:

> Yeah, it has been very stressful. I'll have to admit, though, that I am *relieved*. That this part of it is over, which maybe goes against what I might feel myself about abortion.

> Myself, I just have to get back to some sense of normalcy, if you want to call it that. It is a relief that it's over, that this part's over, and I haven't got the nervous energy to tackle anything else.

> Well, I was relieved after it was done, but I feel bad about it because it was a little life. I think it was the right thing to do, although I'm against abortion, but I think it was.

Seeking Closure

One informant explicitly described her need to find a way to work through the experience of her daughter's pregnancy and abortion and to bring closure to the event:

> I feel some kind of need to write closure to this, and I don't know how to do that. I should feel some sense of relief that it's over with, but there is so much pressure and tension and stress there that I have not been able to bleed it off effectively. . . . I am at a loss to know what it is that I need help with. I haven't identified that for myself yet, like I know what it's *not*. . . . I can tell you what it's not, but I cannot yet tell you what it is. I am going to have to work this through.

Regrouping

Assessing the Outcome

Once the crisis was past, the mothers in this study sought indicators that their daughters had learned a lesson, that they had suffered just a little. Opportunities were provided for the daughters to "talk it out"; but often the daughters did not talk and this was distressing for the mothers. They sought evidence of change as assurance that this would not happen again:

> She never really discussed it with us at all, or even let us know what she was feeling about it, and still hasn't. It was like having a wart removed or something and finding that it was distasteful, but you just got through . . . and things are still no different in that respect. . . . I thought perhaps there might be some kind of emotional . . . well maybe some type of release one way or the other, whether it was crying or really happy or . . . but I don't know there was anything to speak of.

> But she seems to act . . . just like she did before, only difference now is that she is on the pill.

> This suffering [that daughter] is going through right now, she is not going to forget for awhile. And *that's good!* . . . It bothers me to see her suffering like this, but maybe, in her case, maybe it's a good thing that she is feeling a little bit worse than some. But that's good . . . because she has given it a lot of thought, and it has really hit home in her case, so we'll just cross our fingers.

> My biggest concern was that she wouldn't consider it serious enough, that she would take it lightly, because it wasn't . . . it didn't really affect her life all that greatly. That is my concern . . . that she is not going to understand the seriousness of it.

> I don't see any changes. I wish I did.

> It hasn't affected her attitude like I was hoping it would.

Letting Daughter Know Feelings

Two informants said that they had let their daughters know how the experience had affected them:

> I've let her know what it's done to me, too. I've helped her out, you know, a lot before it. I didn't condemn her. I didn't scream at her. Supported her fully, and I knew what she was going through as well, and I didn't even really let her know my thoughts much until after it was over with and she was feeling better which was yesterday, Wednesday, and then when we had the family discussion, I brought out exactly what I felt and let her and my husband know that I was against it totally, you know, and all it would have taken would have been a word. . . . The only reason I went with her

was that's what she wanted. . . . She's only fourteen, and that's what my husband wanted, so. . . .

I can't deny that I have told her that I would not like this, for her to, you know, to make that mistake again.

Postabortion Pregnancy Prevention

The mothers in this study feared another pregnancy could occur; consequently, they are more insistent now about their daughters' contraceptive efforts and because a pregnancy *did* happen they feel they can be more assertive:

I don't think she's questioning the pills. . . . She'll go on whatever contraceptive.

You know, she went through this, and this guy that she knew from before . . . a friend, you know, he phoned her up for a date, and do you know, I did not sleep until she came home. I just could not sleep, I was so afraid. You know, as much as she's told me, "Mom, it won't happen again," you know, I keep thinking will she be forced into this? Now I am so afraid. I don't want her to go out on a date, but I can't do that to her. It's not fair. I have to let her go out. She is a teenager. But I keep thinking Oh my God, will he force her into it, and will it happen again?

She will be on birth control [pills], and hopefully she will remember to take them.

I guess that I just hope she'll be a lot more careful in the future. But we have discussed the idea of an IUD as an alternative because she wasn't always exact about taking them [birth control pills] anyway.

Teaching Other Daughters

Two mothers said they had used the incident of this daughter's pregnancy as an example to other daughters:

We immediately told her little sister about it as well, and we figured that this will be sort of a lesson hopefully learned by the youngest daughter. This is why we made sure the youngest knew everything. We didn't hold it from her, but we hope that she will learn from it.

I did insist that we tell her younger sister, and I did that for two reasons: number one . . . and I told her the reasons . . . I said, "You will need somebody to talk to. You will need somebody at school that you can lean on a little bit," and she was grateful after, and I said, "number two, this is a learning experience for your sister." It was tremendously good for her younger sister. [Daughter] is going to be eighteen next month, and she has a sister who will be seventeen this year. . . . and they [sister and boyfriend] talked about it and decided that she will go on the pill but that they will wait [to have intercourse] until she's been on it for three months because she doesn't want to go through what [daughter] did. So there are some good things that come out of something like this.

Response to the Study

The informants in this study said that it had been therapeutic to talk out their experience with their daughters' abortion:

Well, I think these two talks have done me a lot of good. It was so hard for me to talk. When I said, "murder," that was the first time I'd said it aloud, and I guess once you say it, you feel better. Then you have to convince yourself you're not [a murderer].

It helped me to talk. To let somebody else know how we felt about it, and what we had to go through.

Instead of keeping it in, it's good to let it out.

I was very grateful that somebody did want to hear about it.

Well, I'd like to thank you for the opportunity to tell somebody about it. It helped me, it really has. It is hard to not have somebody to talk to about something like this, particularly somebody that is understanding about it. I think that was one of the hardest things about going through the whole thing is not having somebody . . . you know, somebody that you can tell how you're feeling and get some feedback from them.

Informants' Recommendations

Because the mothers had stated their receptivity to telephone interviewing and that they had appreciated the opportunity to talk out their experience, some informants were asked if they felt a

telephone counseling service would be helpful for families involved
in this crisis:

> It's a marvelous idea. I had to phone to get some information about
> something sort of related to this problem several months ago, and I spoke
> to someone who was a delightful, helpful, empathetic, just a really
> wonderful, warm person to talk to, and when I got off the phone, I felt
> like someone had taken twenty pounds off my shoulders. I think it would
> be a wonderful idea. I think it would be a wonderful service. It's because
> of that fact that nobody knows who's at the end of the phone, and yet
> someone is giving you some advice . . . somebody is telling you that "Hey,
> others have gone through this, you're not alone." Yeah, I think it's a
> tremendously good idea.

> It would be great [telephone counseling] because in so many cases . . .
> you know, personally, I find that when I have a problem I can worry it
> over, and I think I have come up with what is a viable solution, but what
> I actually need to come to a viable solution is to talk it through verbally
> with somebody, and I don't need them to do any more than listen 'cause
> in the process of trying to put it into a way that I can verbalize it, I can
> lead myself to the conclusion. And . . . I can't think that I'm unique in
> that . . . it certainly works for me, and just to be able to do that . . . and
> maybe that is a role that our Planned Parenthood could be fulfilling.

Developing the Model

A salient discovery about the experience of mothers consenting
for their daughters' abortions was that the abortion was not an
isolated event in the lives of the informants and their daughters;
rather, it was part of a comprehensive ongoing process of daughters'
sexual socialization for which the informants had accepted responsibility. This process was both interactive and reciprocal as mothers
and daughters influenced each other. The core category, to which
all other categories were related, was the mothers' acceptance of
responsibility for the sexual socialization of their daughters which
included protecting their daughters from compromising their life
options with an unwanted adolescent pregnancy. This process has
a mother-defined time dimension which begins at the daughter's
birth and continues until the consequences of the daughter's sexual
actions are no longer accepted by the mother, until she sees suffi-

cient indicators of the daughter's competence, or until the daughter assumes the responsibility for herself. This fully variable process, subject to change over time, was identified as a Basic Social Process (BSP) (Glaser, 1978) and labeled *Conducting Daughters' Sexual Socialization* (CDSS).

The core category, CDSS, is made up of three interrelated processes: apprehending, taking responsibility, and evaluating. The first of these, *apprehending,* is defined as a process by which a mother perceives or mentally grasps incipient cues that changes, usually in the daughter's developmental status, warrant a reformation of ideas or strategies employed in CDSS. The bidirectional and contextual influence for change—that is, receiving cues from a variety of sources—is important because it was found in this study that the mothers' apprehension of these cues determined CDSS strategies, and as a result of these cues they reformed their ideas about the situation and the strategies they used to manage it, which also changed the mother-daughter interaction patterns.

The second process, *taking responsibility,* is a broad term which is defined as assuming responsibility for the consequences of the daughter's actions until she is deemed competent enough to act for herself. Intervening is a prominent strategy in this process: that is, the informants attempted to compensate for the developmental, attitudinal, educational, or behavioral deficits which were considered to be compromising their daughters' competence. The informants identified these deficits using the third interrelated process, *evaluating*. Here the informants also integrated and reconciled the events of the CDSS process with their lives and considered the effects on everyone involved in the situation.

Four clear stages in the CDSS process emerged from the data which differentiated and accounted for variations in the informants' behavior, a finding which satisfied one criterion for claiming the discovery of a BSP (Glaser, 1978). During these four temporal stages, pre-pregnancy, pregnancy, abortion, and postabortion, the mothers used different CDSS strategies and these strategy changes influenced behavior in the succeeding stage. That the four stages were indeed, as Glaser (1978) states, "an integrating scheme" (p. 99) that allowed the informants to account for change over time without losing conceptual grasp of the overall process was apparent in that the goal of the informants' purposive action in each stage was the same: to prevent unwanted adolescent pregnancy from compromising their daughters' (and others') life options.

The informants operationalized the conceptual constructs of the CDSS process by employing six major strategies: assessing, informing, being vigilant, accessing services, intervening, and reforming ideas.

The strategy of *assessing* was utilized throughout all four stages and involved being sensitive to cues that their daughters were sexually active, determining that their daughters were pregnant, and evaluating the impact of the abortion on their daughters. A second strategy used by mothers was *informing. Informing* involved sharing information about sexual topics, contraception, and the consequences of adolescent pregnancy. Most of the mothers in this study were aware of the fact that their adolescent daughters would be reluctant to seek information from them; therefore, they took responsibility for assessing their daughter's level of sexual activity and providing appropriate interventions to prevent pregnancy. Those mothers who had not discussed contraception with their daughters had not yet thought of them as sexually active.

Being vigilant was a covert strategy used by the informants and it involved the attentive monitoring of their daughter's behaviors. The informants vigilantly monitored their daughter's menstrual cycles and attempted to monitor boyfriends, friends, and life-styles. *Being vigilant* was a protective device, and through this strategy the mothers in this study allowed their daughters to develop autonomy while keeping a maternal safety net under them.

Accessing services was a fourth strategy used by the mothers in the CDSS. Utilizing this strategy the mothers helped their daughters receive the professional care they needed. This strategy was used to ensure that their daughters received contraceptive counseling, pregnancy testing, and were able to gain access to the abortion procedure.

Intervening was a strategy used by the mothers to protect their daughters. When the mothers in this study suspected their daughters were pregnant they *intervened* by confronting them directly, by involving themselves in the decision-making process regarding the pregnancy, and by consenting for their daughters' abortions.

Reforming ideas was the final strategy used by the mothers in this study. This strategy involved the incorporation of new information and insights and the process of reforming old concepts about their daughters as well as reforming strategies and attitudes to ensure their daughters would not become pregnant again.

Notes

1. Although laws regulating access to abortion change rapidly, at the time this study was done, the host hospital required parental consent for unemancipated women under the age of 18 years to undergo an abortion procedure.

2. A purposive sample of 13 mothers who had consented for their daughter's abortions was selected. To avoid extraneous variables and possible legal implications, mothers whose daughters were pregnant as the result of rape or incest were excluded. The mothers' ages ranged from 32 to 52 years. Eight of the informants were married and living with their daughter's father, two were widowed and were living alone with their daughters, one was remarried and was living with her husband who was not the daughter's father, and two were separated or divorced (one of these mothers lived alone with her daughter, and the other one lived alone and her daughter resided with the father). The daughters ranged in age from 14 to 17 years, and all but two were attending school. All of the abortions took place in a large urban general hospital. Mothers were initially contacted on the day of their daughter's abortion and were asked to participate in the study. Those who agreed to participate were later contacted by telephone.

References

Bernard, J. (1975). *Women, wives, and mothers*. Chicago: Aldine.

Bloch, D. (1972). Sex education practices of mothers. *Journal of Sex Education and Therapy, 7*, 7-12.

Bryan-Logan, B. N., & Dancy, B. L. (1974). Unwed pregnant adolescents: Their mothers' dilemma. *Nursing Clinics of North America, 9*(1), 57-68.

Fox, G. L. (1980). The mother-adolescent daughter relationship as a sexual socialization structure: A research review. *Family Relations, 29*, 21-28.

Glaser, B. G. (1978). *Theoretical sensitivity: Advances in the methodology of grounded theory*. Mill Valley, CA: Sociology Press.

Herold, E. S. (1981). Contraceptive embarrassment and contraceptive behavior. *Journal of Youth and Adolescence, 10*, 233-242.

Herold, E. S. (1984). *Sexual behavior of Canadian young people*. Markham, Ontario: Fitzhenry & Whiteside.

Herold, E. S., & Goodwin, M. R. (1980). Premarital sexual guilt and contraceptive use. *Family Relations, 30*, 247-254.

Herold, E. S., & Way, L. (1983). Oral-genital behavior in a sample of university females. *The Journal of Sex Research, 19*, 327-338.

Jorgensen, S. R., & Sonstegard, J. S. (1984). Predicting adolescent sexual and contraceptive behavior: An application of the Fishbein model. *Journal of Marriage and the Family, 46,* 43-55.

Lindemann, C. (1974). *Birth control and unmarried young women.* New York: Springer.

Marsman, J. (1983). *Mother-child communication about sex.* Unpublished master's thesis, University of Guelph, Guelph, Ontario.

Reiss, I. L. (1973). *Heterosexual relationships inside and outside the marriage.* Morristown, NJ: General Learning Press Module.

Rosen, R. H. (1980). Adolescent pregnancy decision-making: Are parents important? *Adolescence, 15*(57), 43-54.

Rosen, R. H., Benson, T., & Stack, J. M. (1982). Help or hindrance: Parental impact on pregnant teenagers' resolution decisions. *Family Relations, 31,* 271-280.

Scher, P. W., Emans, S. J., & Grace, E. M. (1982). Factors associated with compliance to oral contraceptive use in an adolescent population. *Journal of Adolescent Health Care, 3,* 120-123.

Youngs, D. D., & Niebyl, J. R. (1975). Adolescent pregnancy and abortion. *Medical Clinics of North America, 59,* 1419-1427.

6

The Unrelenting Nightmare: Husbands' Experiences During Their Wives' Chemotherapy

SHARON WILSON

One of the greatest changes to have occurred in the past thirty years in health care is the recognition of patient rights and the rights of the relatives involved in the patient's experience. Whereas in obstetrics the husband has been incorporated into the childbirth experience, in oncology the spouse is paradoxically included and excluded. At one time the spouse was the only person given information regarding the diagnosis, and he or she was urged to keep this information from the patient. More recently, although some information is still kept "behind the scenes" and given only to the spouse, physicians have become more open with patients. Although the spouse's role in supporting the patient is now acknowledged, often the spouse is still made to feel like "the third wheel" in the treatment setting; even so, spouses often suffer during the patient's illness experience. The value of this study is the exploration and explication of the experience of the person closest to a patient undergoing chemotherapy.

One of the hazards of repeated, in-depth, interactive interviews is that the researcher may also become imbedded in the informant's nightmare. How does the researcher listen to such suffering and remain detached? How does the researcher "get inside the mind" of the informant and remain unscathed?

AUTHOR'S NOTE: Derived from: Wilson, S. (1988). *Living with chemotherapy: Perceptions of husbands*. Unpublished master's thesis, University of Alberta, Edmonton, Alberta, Canada.

This research was supported in part by the Alberta Foundation for Nursing Research and the Alberta Association of Registered Nurses.

Cancer represents an abrupt and feared assault on the well-being of the patient and his or her family. Although the response to treatment has improved, the diagnosis of cancer continues to convey a threat of intractable pain, hopelessness, and a prolonged period of wasting away before death (Klagsbrum, 1983). Although new treatment modalities offer some hope, they often produce many adverse effects over which the patient has little control. Increasingly, patients with cancer receive treatment in the form of chemotherapy. Many of these patients receive their treatments on an out-patient basis. Patients and their families must organize their day-to-day lives around the chemotherapy treatments. Although "lip service" is often given to family-centered care, the effects of an individual receiving chemotherapy on the family unit is not well understood.

The cancer experience is stressful not only for the patient, but also for the spouse who is attempting to provide support for the patient. The spouse is often the most important influence on the patient's response to cancer and the side-effects of the treatment (Fernsler, 1986; King & Taylor, 1987). The spouse must also help maintain a normal family life, and as men have traditionally worked outside the home they must make major changes if they are to care for and support their wives while maintaining a semblance of family life. Because a husband can potentially have such an important influence on his wife's responses to chemotherapy and on the quality of life at home, a study was conducted to explore the experiences of husbands during their wives' chemotherapy treatments.[1]

Buffering was a process by which the husbands were able to set up a protective zone around their wives. The *buffering* process (Figure 6.1) was very delicate and the informants had to be constantly reassessing their *buffering* strategies and developing new ones. The assumption underlying the buffering process was that if the husband has a positive attitude toward the outcome of the chemotherapy treatment it will be less stressful for the wife and influence her length and quality of life.

Buffering requires personal attributes such as patience, persistence, understanding, compassion, and a caring marital relationship. It is not a passive role; rather, it involves two active components: constant vigilance and cognitive action. Vigilance consists of watching others and observing the wife's response to chemotherapy and her interactions with others. Cognitive action consists of interpreting these perceptions and then planning an action to *buffer.* Cognitive

Course of illness

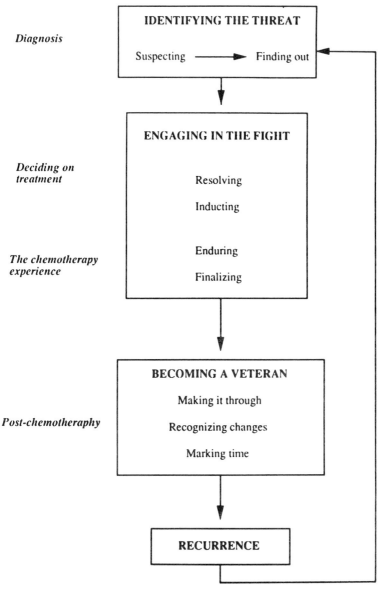

Figure 6.1. The Process of Living with Chemotherapy: Experiences of Husbands

action involves either anticipating or reacting to a situation perceived to be harmful to the wife's well-being.

In order to make the wife's cancer experience less stressful the informants in this study used *buffering* behaviors to reduce or eliminate any potentially harmful threat, to enhance their wives' coping abilities, or to alter their wives' perception of the threat of cancer, thereby making it less harmful. Examples of *buffering* behaviors reducing or eliminating potentially harmful threats were *guarded optimism, second-guessing, taking charge, resisting disruption, treading lightly, omitting the truth, preserving self,* and *orienting to the future.* Examples of *buffering* behaviors that enhanced the wife's coping abilities were *supporting, cherishing, assuming a passive role, maintaining motivation, using humor,* and *orienting.* Examples of *buffering* behaviors that altered the wives' perception of the cancer threat were *making sense, being positive, normalizing, being there, adding on,* and *disguising one's feelings.*

The experience of living with a wife undergoing chemotherapy is a process (Figure 6.2) that consists of three essential components: identifying the threat, engaging in the fight, and becoming a veteran. Not all of the informants in this study proceeded to the fourth component of recurrence, but those who did began the process again. Thus this process is cyclical and repetitive in nature.

Identifying the Threat

The informants in this study said the threat caused by their suspicions that their wives had cancer was ominous. In order to identify and respond to this threat the informants engaged in a process of *suspecting* and *finding out* (see Figure 6.3).

Suspecting

At the beginning of their wives' illness the informants in this study suspected that something was "not right," and they became worried about the well-being of their spouse. Because the informants only suspected their wives had cancer they gathered evidence to support or negate their suspicion. Becoming aware, worrying, and beginning to act were part of this suspecting period.

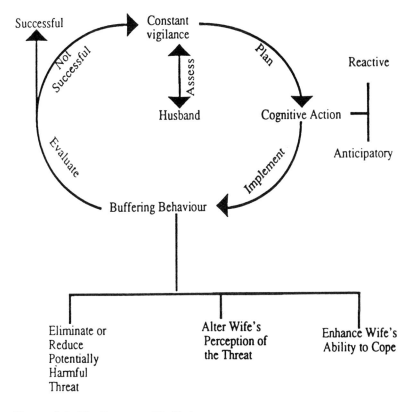

Figure 6.2. The Process of Buffering

Becoming Aware

Although some of the informants were unaware of the abnormal change in their wives' bodies and they were not always advised of a problem by their wives, most of them suspected that something was not right with their wives' health. For example, although no conclusive evidence supported his suspicion, one informant intuitively suspected his wife's problem was cancer. In another case the informant's wife did not want to tell her husband because of his own health problem. During this time the informants encouraged their wives to

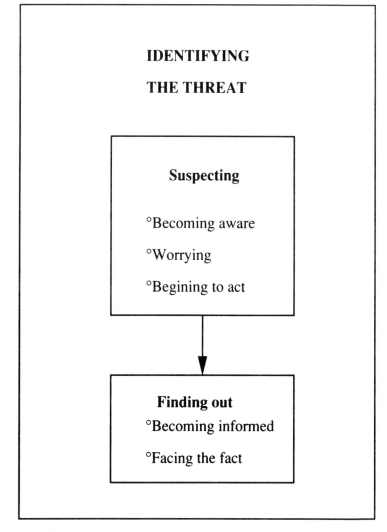

Figure 6.3. The Process of Identifying the Threat

visit a physician and they all expected the problem to be resolved with an easy course of treatment.

Worrying

Initially, the informants believed they did not need to worry and they were convinced not to worry by their wives' responses (particularly when she was a nurse), a previous benign biopsy, and the physician's attitude of "nothing to worry about." Because it had never been encountered before cancer was not often considered as the source of the wives' health problem. The wives' past illnesses had been minor and easily cured and the informants assumed that this would be the case again.

The informants started to worry when they began to have doubts about the gravity of their wives' problem. Doubt was introduced when the physician said she needed a biopsy. For example, the physician met one informant in the hallway just after his wife was taken to surgery and told him that "it did not look good." In addition, doubt and worry increased when the couple received conflicting information regarding diagnosis or when the wives were afraid.

Apprehension and doubt increased while the informants waited for the diagnosis and these fears and doubts created an undercurrent of sadness. In addition to waiting for the diagnosis other situations also aggravated the informants' growing apprehension: the wife's decision to seek another medical opinion, the mention of surgery, or when family members and friends kept asking for news. For example, one informant worried about cancer as soon as surgery was mentioned because his grandmother had worried about cancer before her gallbladder surgery. For another informant the doubt became overwhelming when his wife was sent to see a specialist who practiced in a setting devoted to serving people with cancer.

Beginning to Act

Worrying prompted further responses while the informants waited for the diagnosis. For example, when a physician advocated a "wait and watch" approach one couple became angry and attempted to find a surgeon who was willing to perform a biopsy. Other couples phoned their physician's office for feedback when they felt they were waiting too long for test results:

Waiting for results from the lab was really a torture situation. It was extremely stressful when you suspected very strongly, and yet nobody had come out and said this is what it is. When you're waiting for the phone to ring, you're wondering. It was very stressful waiting to hear. You felt so damn helpless. Phoning didn't seem to help. Nothing seemed to help.

The informants used self-discipline to control their imagination and to avoid thinking about the worst scenario:

It's the unknown, the not knowing, which was the most stressful. It's fear of the unknown; fear of your mind starting to go off in all directions. You imagine all kinds of things. That's where you have to say hold it. You've got to use self-discipline. Say to yourself that you don't know those things, so don't let your imagination start going wild on you. You had to be aware that it was happening in order to control it. It took so long for the diagnosis to be confirmed.

The stress associated with waiting for the diagnosis was so great that one informant required increased medication to avoid aggravating an existing heart condition.

Finding Out

Finding out involved becoming informed of the diagnosis of cancer and facing this fact. This knowledge brought the uncertainty of suspecting to a sudden end:

Now you knew what it was that you had to deal with, you were not guessing. You were not always hoping and at the same time realizing that the hope may be a false hope. You were not going up and down like a yo-yo. Now you were in the drink, and you damn well had to swim. You were not wondering how you were going to cope with it if you happened to fall in the water. You fell in the water, and you found that you were swimming. Now it was a matter of what you had to do to stay afloat and head for shore.

The informants were overwhelmed by the speed with which things happened. Once told about the diagnosis they were thrust "from the frying pan into the fire pretty quick" and they felt they had to make decisions about treatment immediately.

Becoming Informed

Although in one instance the informant had to question his wife in order to learn the diagnosis, usually the informants were advised of the diagnosis of cancer by either their wife or the physician. Sometimes the physician informed the couple together and being summoned to the physician's office was seen as an ominous sign. For example, one physician had his nurse telephone the patient and request that she and her husband come to his office that same evening. The situation was frightening because the wife, a nurse, knew this approach usually meant "bad news." When this informant arrived home from work his wife was overwrought; and even though he felt "totally unprepared" for what was to come he tried to comfort her.

When the physician chose to tell the informant privately about his wife's cancer it was for the purpose of delegating responsibility. For example, the husband was delegated either to inform his wife of her diagnosis, take her to a future appointment, or make sure she was admitted for surgery or treatment. Two informants met with the physician when their wives were not present: One physician met with an informant as he was coming from his wife's surgery to tell him the extent of the disease and to verify that the diagnosis was cancer, and another physician telephoned an informant asking him to come to the hospital where he personally informed him of his wife's diagnosis.

Being informed by phone was helpful for those finding out about recurring cancer. The underlying assumption of the telephone call was that the informant would tell the spouse about the extent of her disease. For one informant this approach allowed him to express his disappointment privately before having to tell his wife, and as a result he felt better prepared "to handle it." He felt he could tell his wife in a more humane manner than the physician because he could tell her when, where, and how he wanted. This approach also allowed him to maintain control of the situation.

In order that the wife would not have to relive the shock with each new telling of the story the informants usually informed children and significant others. The informant's role of informing others helped family and friends get over the initial shock and it also allowed his wife to save her energy.

Determining the extent of the cancer meant enduring a battery of diagnostic tests. For the informants and their wives the unrelenting fear, uncertainty, and shock seemed to last forever and the spouses mirrored each other's anxiety: "I was tense, she was tense. She got tenser from me, and I got tenser from her. We just kind of went around in a circle for a while." Finally, in order to be useful in providing support and strength during the fight the informants decided that they must stop mirroring their wives' responses.

Surgery often occurred very quickly after diagnosis and it was conducted in one of two ways: a biopsy followed by more extensive surgery or one episode of major surgery. The biopsy was conducted either in the physician's office or in the hospital. When performed in a physician's office the patient went home after the procedure to await the results. When surgery was exploratory the informants waited during the operation for news from the physician. Although the informants had confidence in the surgeon, they waited with *guarded optimism* and dreaded hearing the prognosis. *Guarded optimism* was a paradoxical process of preparing for "the worst thing that could happen" while projecting only positive thoughts when with their wives. Even though the informants had *guarded optimism,* the worst scenario (i.e., the wife's death) always lurked in the back of their minds.

Finding out the results of surgery before their wives did gave the informants time to adapt to the situation. Although one informant was delegated to inform his wife, the wives were usually informed of the results of the surgery by the surgeon. After hearing the prognosis the informants were forced to acknowledge their own terror, despair, and sadness. The intensity of these responses required measures designed to "cover up" the depth of their feelings without entirely hiding their response.

Although the wives' hospitalization following extensive surgery offered the informants a reprieve, their wives' hospitalization often distressed the informants. The reality of the situation became obvious for the informants as they watched their wives endure daily equipment and dressing changes. Driving from home or work to the hospital was a quiet period, a time when some informants secretly cried to express their despair.

Facing the Fact

The informants said they experienced fear, helplessness, and "total shock." They were afraid their wives' death was imminent and they described being thrust into a situation where they had no choice: "There was nothing you could do about it." Many of them were unable to cry and one informant said he had not cried since his wife became ill. During this time many of the informants described being emotionally numb "from head to toe":

> The first couple weeks was real shock and despair. Just like someone knocked the wind out of you. You're just totally disillusioned and totally thrown for a loop.

A feeling of uncertainty prevailed and the informants said they felt lost, unbalanced, lacked direction, and did not know which way to turn.

Facing the fact heralded important changes for the informants. One of the informants changed from someone who was emotionless and never talked about himself to someone able to express his feelings more openly, for example showing more compassion for his wife—more than he had for years. Many of the informants reported an increased closeness and strengthening of the marital bond.

After becoming informed the informants asked questions such as: What is cancer? What do I know about cancer?

> The worst nightmare was her succumbing to the disease. The worst nightmare is cancer not being cured and that it metastasizes somewhere else in your body. That's the worst nightmare. Particularly in the wrong place, it's game over. That's the worst nightmare, without a doubt.

For the informants in this study cancer was closely related to death:

> As soon as you hear cancer, it was immediate, that she may die. Not will she die, or not might she die, but when she dies, or how long is this going to go on before she dies?

These thoughts were reinforced when physicians discussed survival statistics or specific survival times. Suddenly forced to recognize that cancer kills, the informants were forced into a life-threatening situation. Not knowing anyone who had cancer or who had survived the disease reinforced the informants' prevailing thoughts of death. The informants had no idea of what to expect or how to begin to cope with such a crisis. They were vulnerable because they felt unable to act maturely and were overcome with grief.

After the diagnosis of cancer was confirmed, the informants began "seeking a cause" for their wives' cancer. The informants considered heredity or family history, diet, stress, smoking, use of the birth control pill, age, previous breast surgery, previous experiences with cancer both within the family and/or within the realm of friendship, excessive use of alcohol or medications, and chance. Younger informants assumed it was a disease restricted to older people. The informants wondered whether they might have caused the cancer. This frightening idea often prevailed for a long time and in some cases it was never definitely discarded. Interestingly, those who had good marriages were most susceptible to this idea of causation and they felt guilty about their presumed role in causing the cancer. These informants felt they could not legitimately rule themselves out as a causative factor when there was no proof of a definite cause: "I'd like to think that I didn't have anything to do with it, that it wasn't my fault, but I wondered."

The informants saw themselves as the more likely victim and they wondered *why my wife and not me?*

> If I expected anybody to get cancer it would be me because I've consumed enough alcohol, have smoked grass. . . . I would be the one that would be more likely to have something like that happen to them.

The informants felt guilty because their wives' cancer was not their disease. Those who had a good marriage began to absolve themselves of the guilt by sharing ownership of the illness and responsibility for the treatment:

> I keep saying we felt, like I guess I feel like this is my disease, too. That's because it's so drastic. It's a fight that she has to undertake, so it's partly mine, too. It's a psychological thing, the helplessness for the husband. This is not just her disease, it is my disease, too.

When informed of the diagnosis after major surgery the informants described feeling unstable and inconsolable. On seeing his wife, one informant became weak, dizzy, and afraid she was going to die. He had no time to pause and reflect because he felt an obligation to inform relatives and family immediately. Seeing his wife's condition and telling others helped this informant face the fact of his wife's cancer and reinforced the reality of the situation.

The informants also became angry, mainly because they felt helpless. For some of the informants the anger was never resolved:

> You feel so damn helpless. You can't buy a cure for her. You can't create a cure for her. It's such a helpless feeling, cancer.

> It troubled me a great deal, the anger, resentment. It's a very mixed-up time, you don't know what your own emotions are. You are going around in circles. You don't know what the hell to think. You don't know what to feel. A very confusing time.

Several informants believed earlier treatment might have influenced the extent of the disease and they were angry at the waiting and the delays prior to diagnosis. Another informant was angry because the frivolity of a new marriage was "taken away." The dilemma was *who could one be angry at?* Because the physician controlled the treatment and the nurse controlled the caregiving, the informants felt getting angry at them might affect the wife's treatment; consequently, the informants got angry at "things," such as the disease or the treatment institution.

Engaging in the Fight

The Canadian Cancer Society widely publicizes a slogan that states "cancer can be beaten." What might this imply to a person and/or family living with cancer? The suggestion that cancer is an entity one can fight and beat indicates that cancer is something one does not want to experience passively. The implication is that cancer can be overcome. This analogy of battling or fighting is something that must ensue *if* one is to win. Thus, fighting is equated with winning. A further implication in the slogan is *if* one fights, *then* one can be hopeful of beating or curing the cancer. Finally, the slogan also places the onus on the *person* to *"do battle"* and *"win"* rather than on the caregivers or the therapy. The demand that one must fight in order to succeed assumes that *if* one works hard enough, *then* one will succeed. When one does not win the fight the blame is not placed on the caregiver or the therapy because the caregiver and the therapy are not fighting the battle. The only ones left to blame are the patient and the spouse. The informants in this study felt they were responsible for identifying "ways" for assisting their wives in beating cancer. As a result of this role the informants felt a responsibility for finding ways to win, and if they did not appear to be winning they felt an overwhelming sense of guilt. As illustrated in Figure 6.4, the informants helped their wives "take on" the fight and were inducted into and endured the chemotherapy. For the informants this fighting process provided hope.

Resolving to Take On the Fight

Resolving to take on the fight involved knowing the diagnosis, achieving a sense of control, crying, and assuming an attitude of *guarded optimism*:

> You've resolved that she has it, and you have to take it on and fight it and try to beat it.

> The shock happened, and then you kind of resolved yourself to the fact that you're just going to have to fight it. You're just going to have to do whatever's necessary—surgery, chemotherapy, radiation. You just get resolved into saying we have to do whatever we can to solve the problem here, so let's go for it.

Admitting to knowing "she has it" did not imply understanding. Understanding came slowly as the informants progressed through the fight and internalized a personal meaning for cancer. Personal meanings were influenced by unresolved anger and the type of marital relationship. Those informants who were possessive of their wives vowed to remain loyal to the fight, whereas those who were angry reacted by being stubborn about giving up and they vowed to help "do whatever's necessary to stay alive."

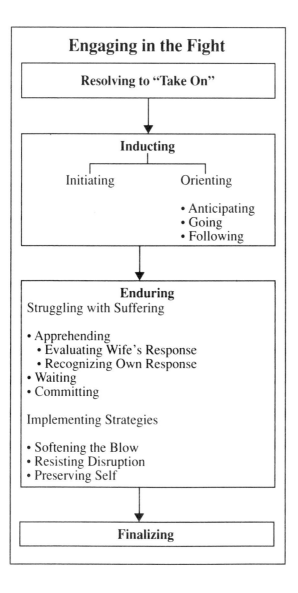

Figure 6.4. The Process of Engaging in the Fight

Realizing the situation was not immediately terminal provided time and motivation for fighting the disease. Resolving to fight provided a sense of control. Participating meant there were things one could do to help even though *guarded optimism* surfaced. "A good cry" often signified the beginning of the resolution to fight. This initial cry represented a means for relieving the shock and expressing sadness. Afterward, the informants felt they had to "get it together" because they felt a sense of responsibility to act for their wife and family.

Inducting

Inducting was the period of time leading up to and including the initial chemotherapy treatment, and it involved *initiation* and *orientation*.

Initiation

Even though the informants were happy to have their wives home with them, *coming home* after surgery was a traumatic experience. Unsure of what was expected, the informants frequently asked what was the right way to act? One of the biggest hurdles of *coming home* postoperatively was the wife's ability to expose her incisional scar. This was especially true after breast surgery and the longer it was deferred the more anxious the informants became. Several inform-ants asked their wives to show them the scar, and many found it was more cosmetically acceptable than expected. One husband said the year following surgery was the most stressful. Factors affecting the informants' stress included financial difficulties incurred when changing jobs, the parental assistance required by young children involved in extracurricular activities, and the informants' inability to decline any request for his time and energy.

The couple decided together or the informant concurred with his wife's decision to accept the physician's suggestions for treatment. Informants usually "played it safe" and did not advocate a treatment that opposed either the physician's or his wife's wishes. The fur-thest any informant ventured was to suggest seeking second and sometimes third opinions from different physicians. One informant wanted his wife to seek further medical opinion and she refused. He felt the need to pursue this and without his wife's knowledge he approached the physician on his own. In return for his concern the informant was severely rebuked by the physician who threatened to withdraw his care. The informant learned abruptly that he could not be a participant in his wife's treatment without jeopardizing the care she received from that particular physician. He also learned not to question any aspect of his wife's medical treatment with the physician. For this informant the lack of information (being kept *"in the dark"*) was the hardest aspect of the entire fight.

Sexual relationships did not resume for some time after surgery. The major influencing factor was the fear of causing the wife further pain and discomfort in the surgical site. When the pain after surgery was severe the couple did not sleep together in the same bed. The decision to sleep in another bed was usually made by the informants because they were afraid of unconsciously hurting their wives while asleep. In particular after breast surgery, it took time to convince the wives that they continued to be sexually attractive:

> I don't know how long it took her to really believe that I still thought she was beautiful, that I was still sexually attracted to her. [It] took her a while to get over that part of the shock.

When the cancer was inoperable the informants said their wives were devastated. This reaction occurred because surgery was perceived to be a more efficient method of treatment than either radiation or chemotherapy. Fear and doubt increased, and when the informants asked the physician why surgery was not an option they never received a satisfactory answer.

How was Treatment Decided?

Alternate methods of treatment (those other than conservative medical methods) were considered, but the time the couples had to learn about these alternatives was limited. When the physician and/or specialist suggested conventional treatment, the informants felt compelled to decide and to begin treatment immediately. The lack of knowledge and the inability to "make the problem go away" compounded the informants' feelings of powerlessness in finding a cure for their wives' cancer. The situation offered the informants no choice but to trust the physicians and to orchestrate what was necessary to solve the problem.

The informants believed the chemotherapy had to work, that it would put the cancer "into check" and allow their wives to live a fairly normal life. Making sense of and rationalizing the treatment were strategies the informants used to deal with the information overload and establish trust in the efficacy of chemotherapy. The informants tended to dwell on statistics when they were advantageous and to compare cancer to other diseases that were incurable or more unsightly in order to make their situation less threatening.

The informants had little knowledge about what chemotherapy was, how it was given, or what effects to expect after the treatment. One informant, who felt anything was better than the statistics for survival without chemotherapy, described "just living in blissful ignorance" before experiencing the first chemotherapy treatment. When chemotherapy was offered as treatment for recurrence of cancer it was accepted immediately. Although the impact of the recurrence of cancer was just as devastating as with the initial diagnosis, the informants had become conditioned to living with the cancer. Chemotherapy represented hope for prolonging life and for curing the disease, and thoughts of "giving up" were intolerable.

Orientation

Orienting to the first chemotherapy treatment influenced the coping strategies used by the informants during subsequent treatments. The first treatment was the time to "learn under fire," and the information gained during the initial chemotherapy treatment helped to decrease the informants' anxiety about the unknown.

Anticipating Chemotherapy

It doesn't compute until you start seeing it happen. You know it just doesn't register. After seeing the first session and seeing everything happen, the [following] ones were a lot easier to cope with because you knew what was going to happen.

Until I actually saw what it was doing, I really didn't have much of an idea.

Although the informants knew the purpose of chemotherapy, they did not know how to respond or what to expect during the first treatment. They wondered but never asked why chemotherapy was not started after surgery (treatment usually began one month after recuperation from the surgery). Side-effects were expected to appear quickly and they were nervously awaited.

The physician was a powerful influence on the husband's outlook, particularly if he was confident chemotherapy would "do the job." *Being positive* did not allow the intrusion of any doubt, and in turn this enhanced the informants' trust and hope in treatment. One informant asked the physician,

> How long has she got to live? He [the physician] said, "Don't you ever ask me that question again because I'm not God. Don't you ever ask me that question again."

This physician's punitive response effectively stopped the informant from asking the question again, even after several recurrences of his wife's cancer. The informant's response was not one of anger but one that accepted the physician's directive.

Going to Chemotherapy

Accompanying their wives to the initial chemotherapy treatment was a monumental decision for the informants in this study. This decision was influenced by the wife's request for his presence, his own personal need to understand the treatment, and the informant's health, work commitments, and familiarity with the treatment facility. A sense of foreboding and death was associated with cancer and the informants were aware of the need to resolve this attitude before they could be of assistance to their wives.

The informants' initial learning experiences were varied because everything was new. The informants looked for the "norm" or "the right thing to do" as they became familiar with the rituals associated with going to chemotherapy. They asked questions and watched how their wives responded to the treatment facility and the treatment, what other husbands did during treatment, how the chemotherapy was given, and how the physician and nurses interacted with patients and families. They noted other patients, particularly their ages, skin color, and whether or not they had experienced hair or weight loss. The informants felt alien in a world where their wives belonged. Other patients stared at them, the nurses did not talk to them, and often there were no other husbands present. This experience reinforced the informants' need to adapt to their wives' situation and it highlighted the life threatening aspects of the situation.

The response to the treatment facility was varied and often reflected anger toward the disease or previous treatment. Many of the informants initially hated the treatment facility, although others were pleasantly surprised to find that the patients and health care personnel were friendly, ordinary people. The informants expected the other patients to look sad, depressed, or very ill, but these expectations were not fulfilled. Also, long periods of inactivity were not uncommon while waiting for treatment, and the informants began to appreciate waiting as an integral part of chemotherapy.

Following Chemotherapy

Coming home after the chemotherapy treatment involved filling prescriptions and then waiting for something to happen. The informants did not respond to the initial chemotherapy experience until their wives were resting in bed, and they said that during this period they lacked time, energy, and mental awareness. In one case, the initial experience was devastating as the wife experienced extreme side-effects immediately after coming home. The informants watched to determine how long their wives were ill following treatment, when the illness began and subsided, and when their wives began to feel good again. They watched their wives when they thought their vigilance was not noticed and they tried to predict their wives' needs. There was little they could do for their wives and many felt clumsy, helpless, and in the way as they hovered around their wives. The need to help competed with the need to protect their wives' privacy. One informant found himself in a decision-making role as he tried to decide whether or not to call the physician when he thought his wife's illness was severe.

Wives read voraciously about cancer and the informants tried to keep up with their wives' reading. Discussion about this reading was ongoing between the spouses and it served to bring the couple closer together. Basically, the informants read to find a cure.

The informants spent increasing amounts of time with their wives, often excluding friends and family. Several of them took early retirement or simply quit their jobs. The focus of daily life was the wife's needs, which was particularly difficult for those informants who continued to work because they had to divide their time between work and home.

At this time, the informants assumed a *doer* role. The *doer* role enabled the informants to receive feedback for caring tasks, and because they were often unable to talk about their concerns without crying, *doing* allowed the informants to physically express their concern for their wives. In addition, the informants felt guilty discussing their own feelings when they knew their wives were going through a much worse experience. Taking a submissive position was something the informant believed was necessary even though it perpetuated the guilt he felt for being healthy. The informants believed their wives wanted them to be strong and in control of their feelings. As a result, most of the informants tried to hide the intensity and depth of their feelings by being quiet and supportive.

Enduring

Enduring involved dealing with the side-effects caused by the chemotherapy treatment. *Enduring* included struggling with suffering and implementing strategies designed to buffer. Figure 6.5 depicts how the quality of the marital relationship influenced the strategies the informants used to fight and endure the side-effects of chemotherapy.

Those informants who enjoyed a good marital relationship were active participants and shared the cancer experience with their wives. They accepted the disease as "their disease," were empathetic to their wives' suffering, and emphasized "being positive" (Figure 6.5, Cell *a*). Those informants who were in a poor marital relationship stayed to help their wives but they were not hopeful of curing the cancer. They respected the decision making of others and abided by the desires of their wives (Figure 6.5, Cell *b*).

Those informants who had a good relationship but indulged in self-pity were convinced their wives could not endure the fight without their presence. They were skeptical about chemotherapy as a cancer treatment and their outlook was not overly positive. They made their wives dependent by taking over for them (Figure 6.5, Cell *c*). Those informants who said they had poor marriages felt no commitment or compassion toward their wives and took no responsibility for supporting them during treatment. These men eventually left their wives because the situation became too difficult to endure

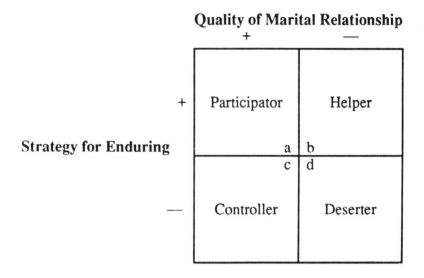

Figure 6.5. The Relationship Between the Quality of the Marital Relationship and the Strategy of Enduring

and some of them formed a relationship with someone else (Figure 6.5, Cell *d*).

Struggling with Suffering

The purpose of *enduring* the fight was always for the benefit of the wife who had cancer. Struggling was described as:

> When you're thrown into a pool and you can't swim, and you don't have a life preserver, that's the way I felt for a long time. In other words, struggling. It was hard to get up in the morning knowing that you were going to have another one of those days which was unpredictable.

> The bottom line was that you're going to get chemotherapy, you're going to get sick, and hopefully it's going to help you extend your life. You suffer for two and a half days once a month, and you play the numbers game, whereby two and a half days in a month might give you a little longer to live.

> The pain of watching somebody that you love going through pain, going through agony, that is the hardest part. That is the hardest part of the whole thing to deal with that. That was my hardest part—it wasn't the caring, or the cleaning up, or helping her to the washroom, or getting the pills.

> It sort of hits you when the person that's beside you gets sick, has never been sick, and goes through chemo, and comes home and vomits, and holds her teeth in her hand. You start seeing a person so differently. You know, you have to help them to the washroom because they're dizzy. Then you really get to love somebody beyond their physical being.

One informant also described struggling when the disease was progressing:

> It was hell on wheels watching her go downhill. Hardly being able to talk and eat. Just wasting away in front of your eyes, and in really terrible pain. There didn't seem to be much they could do about it.

Struggling involved apprehending, waiting, and committing. The struggle permeated life and indulging oneself was impossible because "the only trouble was she had it and I didn't." Some of the informants became obsessed with the struggle.

Apprehending the Struggle

The informants assessed struggling by being vigilant of their wives' responses to chemotherapy. Evaluating the wife's response and one's own response to chemotherapy comprised apprehending.

Evaluating Wife's Response to Chemotherapy Treatment

Examining beliefs. The informants in this study held several beliefs about their wives' chemotherapy experience. The informants felt they could not have endured the chemotherapy as well as their wives. They said their wives were stronger, tougher, and more resilient, particularly in relation to pain and patience. The informants said they would have been more demanding and despairing in a similar situation, and they felt their wives had a more understanding nature and were more nurturing. One informant felt that he "would find it much harder to be that positive about myself than I am about her." Also, the informants felt they would not make good patients: "[The] littlest thing that goes wrong with me is a major crisis."

Grieving. Even though the wives seldom expressed a fear of dying, by watching their wives grieve the informants were forced to realize that the situation was life-threatening. The informants said their wives began reading obituaries in newspapers and some of the wives arranged their own funeral. One wife introduced the subject of death by warning her husband that 40% of spouses die within a year following their wives' deaths. He said, "This hit me like a ton of bricks. I just shut right up. She was telling me that she was going to die." Although he perceived her concern for him, the consideration of her potential death was too overwhelming for him to consider. Another wife slowly shifted the household and family responsibilities onto her husband as she prepared for her impending death.

Second-guessing. Second-guessing was putting yourself in the other person's position in order to understand his or her experience. The informants found this technique helped them to be

> much more conscious of some of the things that I think I do, or I want to do, or that I do unconsciously. I try to be a little more conscious about what I'm doing, to be more supportive. I try to put myself in my wife's position and ask the question: What would I want me to be like if I were her?

If nurses or physicians were unavailable to answer questions the informants found it difficult to refrain from asking their wives for information. The dilemma was that one always wondered if one was right. *Second-guessing* involved being empathetic and perceptive while recognizing it was impossible to do everything that would please his wife. One informant became aware of forcing his own joviality when what his wife really wanted was privacy; consequently, *second-guessing* helped the informants to be less intrusive.

Changing in response to chemotherapy. The intensity of "being ill" was dependent on the type and dosage of drugs. As chemotherapy progressed, the struggle was more difficult for those whose wives were not improving. Changes in physical appearance became more obvious and included changes in weight, skin color, and texture; gums became tender in the mouth; and "puncture marks" or bruises appeared on the wives' arms. Changes brought the informants back to reality and the wives were described as looking very sad and debilitated. One informant knew his wife suffered terrible "pain in her arms from being tortured so damn many times, her arms were just like a pin cushion." It made him extremely sad to see that his wife "would not wear short sleeves, she kept her arms covered because she did not want to be seen that way." Some of the wives developed a constant body odor. The most unpleasant changes mentioned were those associated with temperament, hair loss, fatigue, and nausea.

The "chemo crazies." The informants were amazed at the rapidity with which their wives' moods would change. While watching this as well as recognizing the loss of their wives' sense of humor, the effects of the drugs became obvious to the informants. One informant described his wife as a "Jekyll and Hyde" because she would scream one minute and be compassionate the next. At one point he had to hit her to "bring her out of her hysteria."

During chemotherapy the informants expected depression, but not the depth of depression experienced by their wives. Moods swung "up and down like a yo-yo," and the informants were unprepared for their wives' extreme mood changes. Wives cried easily and were emotionally frail. One informant, who did not believe his wife was in a life threatening position, could not justify her behavior and became very angry, while another informant labeled his wife's behavior the "chemo crazies." The physical effects would come and go but the "mood swings were always there." When the informants were tired, these side-effects were "very hard to handle." Patience and understanding were needed and the informants tried not to "hate" their wives or "hold a grudge." Some of the informants felt exploited; others said, "She was just venting frustration at the one closest to her." One wife announced her intention to think only of herself, which hurt her husband because he thought he was already putting his wife first. The informants did not argue or say anything in response to their wives' mood changes, and they would "back away" or "accept it" because mood swings "were not her fault."

Losing hair. The informants did not think hair loss was the worst side-effect of the chemotherapy treatment, but they did believe that "losing hair was a major trauma" for their wives. Although hair loss was something the informants had to adapt to and accept, waiting for the event was more stressful for them than seeing their wives without hair. The informants said their wives' major concern was to appear normal. Often the informant was the only person to see his wife bald. Some of the informants were afraid their wives' hair loss was permanent. Others said, "The fact that she lost her hair, well it's not very nice, but it's not the end of the world. It's going to grow back." This attitude was reinforced if they had talked to other women undergoing chemotherapy. Hair loss was a very personal matter that was not discussed with others and the informants resented the question "Has she had any hair loss yet?" Hair loss meant "powerful" drugs were working and this fact consoled some husbands because not all drugs were powerful enough to cause hair loss.

The informants said their wives were horrified by their hair loss, and the wives closely watched their husbands' responses. Many women lost hair all over their body and the informants said they described themselves as "feeling neutered" or feeling "like a eunuch." Sometimes humor was used to counteract the sadness of hair loss, but often the informants' laugh was hollow.

Fatigue. Weight loss due to nausea or a lack of appetite made the wives appear drawn and fatigued. When the informants saw their wives with makeup on, their hair done, and dressed to go out, they sometimes forgot that their wives had limited stamina. Social events became quite infrequent as wives did not feel like "doing anything."

The informants realized their wives were dependent on them and they responded by staying at home, which for some was confining. Some of the informants described this situation as "living alone," even though they felt relieved when their wives slept: "If she's sleeping, she's obviously getting better." The informants said it was necessary to be quiet when their wives were sleeping because any noise caused them to wake up. Some of the informants endured "sleepless nights" although others slept soundly. Although some of the wives needed sleeping pills, the informants did not want their wives taking more medication than required. One wife did not reveal her need for sleeping pills and the husband was angry at being kept *in the dark.*

Nausea. Most of the informants found it difficult to watch and listen to their wives' nausea. One informant described his wife's nausea as "bloody hell" because there was often no respite between treatments. The informants said that their wives' nausea and lack of appetite persisted after the vomiting stopped, and because the wives were concerned about their appearance the informants were constantly trying to preserve their wives' self-esteem during their bouts of nausea:

> She didn't want me to see her without her false teeth. It used to break my heart. I wanted to scream. I just wanted to yell because to see that—her worrying about me—that's the hardest part.

Most of the wives wanted to be alone in the washroom when nauseated or vomiting, although others found their husbands' presence comforting. The informants felt "impotent" because they were delegated to an observer role in the home. They worried about their wives choking, and they were afraid to leave the home:

> It's a terrible thing when you start getting out of the liquid vomit into the dry heaves. It's even worse [because] you just sit there, and what can you do? It's just a helpless feeling—it's just a terrible, helpless feeling.

For some of the wives driving sometimes induced nausea. Frequently vomiting began during the drive home after treatment, which necessitated a receptacle for use in the car. Although one exceptional wife had learned to control her nausea through mind control, for most of the wives the nausea progressed quickly to a state described as being "violently ill, [with] no control [over] the throwing up and the gagging and the nausea." For many of the wives, it was days before they were able to "operate on their own." Although marijuana was sometimes helpful, the medication used to counteract the nausea was ineffective. Wives who were not violently ill were considered lucky and fortunate. One informant administered injections to control the vomiting, which were minimally beneficial.

The wives' inability to eat also worried the informants and they felt guilty preparing food for themselves when the odors associated with cooking or the noise of a closing door could precipitate nausea. For many of the informants the nausea was depressing because "it brought reality right home, right now. It's not hidden. She's sick, there's just no two ways about it." Many of the informants worried that their wives were losing the "fighting spirit" and that they were "almost ready to give up." For increasingly longer periods after the nausea subsided, although their wives "would not really say," the informants "could tell [they were] not feeling good."

Fighting. The motivation and determination to fight were reinforced for those informants who had been told by the physician that their wife "did not have too much time to live." The informants were proud of their wives' determination, fortitude, and strength: "She seemed to have lots of fight in her. She was bound and determined it wasn't going to get the worst of her, and she carried on." When extra medication was required the informants wondered how their wives could possibly "take it." The informants admired their wives' acceptance of.the needles, the "poison," and the effects of the chemicals: "I never figured that she [could] take [that] much abuse. . . . She always looked so sad." In spite of the side-effects of the chemotherapy treatment most of the informants believed their wives never seriously considered discontinuing treatment or ending their own lives.

Supporting. The informants assumed a *supporter* role and learned to accept the situation because their wives were "so good." Some of the informants said they felt little need to be in the home because their wives preferred to "suffer in silence" and did not "want me to be around that much." Other informants were forced to recognize the enormity of the situation when normally independent wives suddenly became dependent. Most of the informants recognized that their wives were doing their best to endure the chemotherapy, often with no hope of avoiding side-effects. It was difficult for the informants to project hopefulness when sadness permeated their thoughts. Others felt hopeless when they thought their wives were giving up the fight: "It was very hard to see my wife in that condition knowing that she was accepting [everything]. I believe she had, in a sense, accepted her fate."

The informants watched but did not interfere with their wives' coping strategies. This passive role enabled the informants to observe their wives' coping strategies without interfering and to focus on "what she wants." This role allowed the informants to plan and implement their own strategies. For those wives who were employed, work interests provided a distraction and a reason to endure and learn to live with the cancer experience, although those wives who did not work or who were unable to work had more time to "worry [and] brood about it more."

Several of the informants said their wives withdrew into a "sick world" which separated them from the "healthy world" of the husband. Recognizing this withdrawal helped the informants appreciate the depth of fear and need for protection experienced by their wives. Many of the informants felt the lack of communication between these two "different worlds" kept them *in the dark,* and they wondered if they were being punished for being healthy.

Going to treatment was traumatic for the informants because their wives "hated" chemotherapy: "She'd rather not go, and she would be silent during the trip to the treatment facility." Some of the wives were "fanatical" about getting to treatment on the exact day, which often became more flexible as time progressed and treatments became more routine. When treatments were postponed the informants' positive attitude was overwhelmed by fear. Although positive thinking was an effective coping strategy (it enabled the informants to think they were in control of the situation), the informants were afraid that the setback caused by a missed or postponed treatment would affect their ability to fight.

The informants were often surprised when their wives talked about the cancer experience in detached, depersonalized clinical terms. The informants felt that talking about feelings was emotionally upsetting and depleted their wives' energy, while the fear of death made it "hard on a person." The informants thought talking about feelings created a "poor me" attitude, which they found appalling. The informants noticed that their wives stopped crying at some point during the course of the chemotherapy treatments, and as a result the wives had no other outlet for expressing fear. Also, the wives often wanted to do things that worried the informants. For example, some of the wives wanted to continue driving a car but the informants were afraid that the chemotherapy might have residual effects which could potentially cause an accident.

Recognizing His Own Response to Treatment

Expressing love. The informants in this study did not initially recognize the enormity of their wives' need to feel loved, and when they did express their feelings of love they were surprised when their wives said they needed to hear it more. Although the most intimate time for expressing love is usually in the privacy of the bedroom, some of the couples did not sleep together and as a result they lost this opportunity to share their love. Many of the wives were up nightly and some of the informants said that this activity disturbed their sleep. Initially, the informants stayed awake during the night but as the treatments progressed those informants who worked were forced to sleep.

Expressing suffering. The informants' reluctance to legitimize their own suffering was evident in this study: "I really don't like to see her suffer. I just have a difficult time handling that, but you handle it." One informant measured himself by his wife's response: "If she felt good, I felt good." In effect, he mirrored her experience:

> When she was suffering with her cancer, in her bad times, I felt pretty bad too. And when she rallied, was feeling good, was cheerful, it seemed as though I was too.

The submissive position the informants assumed served to hide their own suffering and placed less stress on their wives:

> When things bothered me, I suffered in silence. I accepted it, and I dealt with it alone. But only in matters that affected my wife and I.

Creating emotional turmoil. When ongoing treatment did not appear to alleviate their wives' suffering, the informants felt helpless and they began to despair:

> It was extremely difficult to see what was happening to my wife as a result of the chemistry. It was terrible. There was not a damn thing you could do about it. It was really horrendous. It's a horrible experience. I hate to think of what it was like for her.

> I'd rather have suffered it myself. If I could of taken the drugs for her, I would have done it.

The uncertain outcome of chemotherapy magnified the informants' feelings of helplessness: "Her life was constantly threatened. It wasn't as though she was out of the woods." When intense side-effects did not occur the informants often became pessimistic, and they wondered when the side-effects would start and if their wives would be able to endure them.

Although the informants said it was difficult to watch their wives' pain, the sight of a needle, and their wives' injections, they felt the thoughts of their wives' future pain had been more difficult to deal with than the "real pain." The informants recognized the drain on their own energy and they were horrified by the idea of the physical and emotional trauma their wives must be enduring: "I felt a lot of sorrow for her. It is extremely hard to explain when you love somebody and watch them go through agony or turmoil in their mind." After five consecutive days of treatment, one informant had to help his wife bathe and dress to prepare for treatment and he became exhausted because he continued to work. The informants were frustrated with their lack of control and their inability to solve the problem of chemotherapy:

> When you're right in the middle of those treatments, you really can't see the light at the end of the tunnel it seems. And then it becomes a big problem.

For example, missing a treatment due to low blood counts was discouraging and the imagined effect of missing a treatment led the informants to ask "Would the cancer proliferate? Would the wife bounce back and reestablish physical defenses to enable the next treatment?"

Living day-to-day became more important. Taking full advantage of each day was the rule. *If* the wife felt well, then it was a good day; *if* the wife did not feel well, then so be it. As the informants accepted and learned to live with the lack of choice they realized that one could not make "all things better": "You have no choice, you simply just do the best you can." The informants learned to trust that "they [medical personnel] are doing everything they can" to help. It became easier to say "whatever is going to happen, I let happen. I don't try and fight it too much." This attitude allowed the informants to move from fighting the inevitable to using their energy constructively. Short-term goals such as planning for holidays were the only future plans made as long-term goals became nonexistent.

Fear and sadness were always evident: "You're always scared. I was always afraid. Deep in your mind, you knew she wasn't going to get well, and you were so afraid of that." For some of the informants repressing anger conserved energy, although others realized that anger was destructive if it was not expressed: "It could get me down." Often there was no one with whom to express this anger. For some of the informants the physical expression of anger was the only outlet; for example, they broke doors or put their fists through walls. Inanimate objects were always the focus of abuse. Other informants were able to find a private place to yell or scream, but many of them felt they did not have the time for this expression of anger. Instead, the energy expended in expressing anger and resentment was rechanneled into "making sense" of the situation, which was more conducive to helpful behavior. Most of the informants "never got rid of the anger" and never accepted the disease because if one accepted the disease then hope was gone. When hope was gone then one gives up the fight, and this was not acceptable to the informants.

For many of the informants their sadness could not be hidden and they became confused because their sadness was not directed toward any one particular loss. Sadness often produced tension, anxiety, frustration, and physical illness because it was ongoing and relentless. Tears would often be the result of sadness. The informants were sad for their wives, their families, and themselves, and they tried not to let sadness overwhelm them and cause depression or affect their ability to fight.

Changing life-style. Chemotherapy forced a change in life-style and became the focus of daily living:

> It filled our lives. Chemo took a lot of your life. The pills after the being sick, then worrying about going back the next time. I guess that's all part of it.

Life-styles changed to the point where they were described as "not normal":

> It seemed like just the time that she got everything back to what you'd call normal, where she's got her appetite, then it's time for the chemo again.

For some of the informants, every treatment was "always so different, so new," although others felt their wives had about a "week of good health, relatively speaking" between treatments. Changing social

patterns left some informants feeling isolated, although others deliberately isolated themselves. Many of the informants wanted to socialize more but they could not because their wives were "quite often
sick" or "she didn't want to." Sometimes after socializing, wives
became ill with nausea and vomiting and as a result the informants
were reluctant to socialize because of the negative consequences
socializing might hold for their wives. The principle of consequence
also applied to holidays. Chemotherapy was scheduled to accommodate holidays, which gave the wives an "extra week of holidays."
However, on returning home, "she had to pay for it" because treatments were scheduled closer together until she had made up the
missed treatment.

The informants were not prepared for the sudden change in their
life-style:

> You had to change your life-style a whole bunch. On those days you
> obviously couldn't plan on going out. You had to be around to take care
> of your wife.

Although treatments became routine, the unpredictability of the
wife's response to treatment was disrupting. Chemotherapy "took up
so much of your life," and some of the informants wondered if the
physician realized how much chemotherapy required of one's life
because the sickness lasted day and night, often with no period of
reprieve for days. For some of the informants a reprieve never
occurred because the chemotherapy was constantly "on their mind."
For those informants who worked, time was at a premium: "Your life
is so full at the time, between my wife and work, there wasn't spare
time to do anything else."

All of the informants were aware of the passage of time and many
of them became "calendar watchers," admitting "it's terrible to live
to a calendar." The calendar dominated daily living and it was
something one could use to normalize life and "keep track of what
was going on." Although the actual daily response to treatment was
consistently unpredictable, the informants could determine how
many days the sickness would last. For many of the informants it was
difficult to believe the drastic change from being well before the
treatment to the illness following treatment and back to being well
again after the initial effects of the drugs had passed. The day of
treatment was dreaded and it was important to plan ahead:

You just knew that you were going to be home all weekend. Your wife was going to be awfully sick. There's not a heck of a lot you can do about it. There's a reason for this, so just hang in there.

For the informants, "a reason" (fighting the cancer) legitimized staying home.

The informants eventually "settled into the chemotherapy itself" and became resigned to the reality of chemotherapy: "I have to a certain extent gotten used to the fact that she's sick all the time—kind of try to cope with it." One informant coped by "taking care of [himself] and going out, doing things, more than [he] had before." The informants said that sexual relations decreased as the chemotherapy progressed and many of them felt this was due to the fact that their wives had lost interest in them. They had difficulty discussing this with anyone, especially their wives, and most often their concerns were never resolved.

The informants learned to be prepared for their wives' refusal to go to treatment, which was considered a natural reaction to something so unpleasant. Some of the informants felt compelled to make sure their wives went to treatment. For example, one informant said he had to be "blunt" and "insulting" before his wife would agree to go to chemotherapy treatments. Most of the informants felt anxious when their wives said "I want to die" because they felt this meant their wives were giving up. At this point the informants assumed the role of protector:

I've always been very protective of my family. If I could relieve them going through any problems, I would. I would try to solve them, try to shield them.

Also, the informants said they found it difficult to tolerate other members of the family. Children were often described as demanding, self-centered, uncaring, and inept at accomplishing household chores. For younger informants, parents were supportive and helpful; whereas for older informants parental influence was not helpful because they had their own established methods of coping, and they considered parents outsiders. Grandchildren often became important and one couple moved closer to their grandchildren.

Personal coping strategies varied. The informants used excessive eating, smoking, and/or drinking in order to cope, but if these excessive habits were noticed, other ways of coping were devised so that their wives would not worry. Some of the informants read the obituaries, in particular the age and cause of death, although others avoided this "like the plague." When the cause of death was not noted the informants looked for the recipient of contributions in order to determine the cause of death. One informant ingested some of his wife's medication in order to understand what she was enduring. Many of the informants were surprised by their ability to change: "You think you know yourself well, but you really don't until the actual thing happens to you." The informants said they learned to be flexible, which enabled them to become "a better person." The informants felt it was important that something good come out of the experience and they took better care of themselves and their wives.

Relating to others. Few informants attended group support meetings because they were not at ease discussing their personal problems with strangers. Those who did attend these meetings felt they did "not receive" as much as they gave to others. The informants felt the meetings had a self-consoling, poor me attitude which did not support their coping strategy of positive thinking.

The informants felt relatives and friends gave too much support to their wives, which they felt made their wives feel like invalids and intruded on the informant's *doer* role and the couple's privacy. Although people did not always know what to say, most of the informants took strength from the caring and the prayers that were offered on their behalf. For some of the informants old friends were lost and new friends were gained because their wives were not always receptive or amiable. The informants felt acquaintances, those who were not considered friends, often used avoidance strategies because they did not know how to respond or were afraid of the emotional response they might receive. When acquaintances did say something, the informants found that "some will come and talk with me, sort of like a bereavement, as if your wife had died." Many of the informants were frustrated by the question that seemed to open most conversations: "How is your wife?" And they were annoyed that the answer "no change" never seemed to be enough. Rarely did anyone ask informants how *they* were doing.

Maintaining health. Once the informants recognized they were experiencing stress they no longer took their health for granted, and

they worried that if they got sick they would jeopardize their wives'
health. The informants compared their illness to that of their wives'
and realized to watch someone suffer was to hope you did not have
to endure the same experience:

> I used to feel guilty about saying to myself thank God it isn't me. I surely
> wasn't glad that it was my wife. That guilt was really hard to shake or
> understand.

Being informed. Initially the informants questioned the amount
of knowledge they needed to have: "The more you read, the more
frightening it becomes." "Finding a happy medium" was ideal. Later
the informants were grateful they knew and were familiar with the
terminology because it helped them to converse intelligently with
others. Becoming knowledgeable also helped them rationalize and
accept behavioral changes in their wives. For some the acquisition
of knowledge was like a staircase: the more knowledge gained, the
more aware they became of future eventualities. If cancer recurred
the staircase became shorter. Those whose wives were enduring the
recurrence of cancer were treated as "experts" because their experience of climbing this particular staircase was something others had
not encountered.

The informants often felt *"in the dark"* in terms of the information
they received from either the physician or their wife. For example,
some of the informants did not understand continuing chemotherapy when there was no indication of improvement. Those who
accompanied their wives during the physician's examination saw
themselves as more knowledgeable than those who waited outside.
Wives were often uncommunicative after seeing the physician, and
the informants were reluctant to ask them questions. When they did
ask they usually received the standard reply, "Oh nothing." Sometimes the wives would not allow their husbands to be present during
the examination and they wondered why. Was she deliberately
keeping information from him? Was she punishing him for being
healthy?

The informants were told by their wives not to ask too many
questions, so they would often ask a nurse when their wives were
not present. Unfortunately, the nurses were often noncommittal and
noninformative. Most of the informants had no contact with the
physician, believing the physician was too busy to disturb. Being *in*

the dark made the informants feel vulnerable. When wives were not sharing feelings, then how could the husbands? The informants felt they had to withhold their concerns from their wives and this silence was stressful. Sometimes the informants supported their wives when they sought counseling services, but they were not willing to seek help for themselves because the wife was the ill one. Over time the informants learned to live with being *in the dark*.

Orienting to the future. Considering possible outcomes (an aspect of accepting) forced the informants to think about the future. The informants preferred to live day-by-day in order to stay positive and deal with reality and they planned for the future secretively, rarely discussing the future with anyone. Although this secrecy offered comfort and security some of the informants felt guilty, as if this planning for the future meant they were giving up and admitting their wives were not going to get well. Recurring disease often hastened *orienting to the future*; however, some of the informants were unable to orient to the future because they found the idea of death as shocking as the initial diagnosis. These informants were unable to tolerate thoughts of dying, and they "shrugged them off" and never accepted the cancer experience.

Facing the fact involved understanding that the cancer experience was terminal while remaining positive: "Hopefully, it won't be for a long time." The informants knew "the day was coming" when chemotherapy would be ineffective and stopped. Although they dreaded this moment and often experienced a "terrible sense of doom" as the disease progressed, they acknowledged that their life would not end when their wives died. They had to plan for the time following their wives' death because when the time came they might be overwrought and unable to act coherently.

The informants felt sad at the thought of their wives' death and guilty for having these thoughts because their wives were still alive. As a result, many of them continued to think only of a short-term future: "I know next year will be better" or "I think I can tolerate her [behavior] for another four months." Others were unable to fathom anything beyond daily living. Those who witnessed their wives receiving life-support measures were more apt to talk about the future. The physician who told an informant that he "needed to think of his life too" freed him to think of the future without the accompanying guilt.

Preparing for the worst scenario included considering questions such as were wives going to become sicker and die? Although colleagues, friends, or family members suggested that the informants talk to their wives about death, they usually refused to discuss issues associated with dying until the wife initiated the conversation. The informants felt maintaining a positive attitude was essential for their wives' well-being. Discussing the *worst scenario* while undergoing treatment was the same as speculating about death, which the informants felt would neutralize hope for recovery. Some of the informants thought they "should" discuss death with their wives, and they wondered if avoiding the subject meant they were denying the possibility of death. Their answer was no. They acknowledged the existence of the cancer, *but* they had doubts about the future: "I know it's there. I know that it could be deadly. But we'll deal with that when we have to." Therefore, not discussing death with their wives was both a *buffering* behavior and a shared coping strategy.

Talking openly about the future facilitated the acceptance of death. Some of the informants felt justified planning for the possibility of their wives' death when wives completed wills or checked out existing insurance policies, although others became agitated by these actions because they felt it meant their wives were giving up the fight. Most of the informants did not want to consider losing their wives to cancer, and preparing for the worst scenario involved planning: "What will I do?" Many of the informants felt guilt-ridden considering the question of death, and they "blocked it out"; however, it kept reappearing, demanding consideration.

Planning for later illness included concerns about the wives' comfort and pain. The informants began to think about accommodating their wives' wish to remain in the home by considering financial costs, nursing care services, and home management aspects. Unfamiliar with caring for someone in settings other than an acute care hospital, the informants experienced a fear of the unknown while trying to be practical. The informants' major concerns involved carrying on with their job, managing the home, helping children respond to their mother's illness, and finding caregivers who could alleviate their wives' physical suffering. The informants' greatest comfort was to look to others who had survived the fight.

Although the presence of young children made long-term planning necessary, planning for after death usually consisted of short-term goals. The informants said they felt lonely when they thought about the future, and they used coping mechanisms such as "working twice as hard to fill the void" in order to deter these feelings of loneliness. Daydreams, which offered fantasy, relaxation, and enjoyment, were curtailed because of the guilt and the "almost morbid feelings of enjoying themselves." Daydreams included marrying again, where they would live, what they would be doing, and how their family would cope with their wives' death.

Waiting

The waiting game was timeless, fluctuating with the "ebb and flow of the disease":

> The whole thing was a waiting game for me—waiting for results, waiting to see if there was any improvement, waiting to see if she was getting worse, waiting for the end of the chemotherapy. It went on and on and on.

Waiting was ongoing and endless unless one wanted to consider death an acceptable end. Waiting was a passive activity and it frustrated the informants because they were *doers* who felt comfortable problem-solving and acting. The informants waited for their wives to get ready for treatment, for a parking place at the treatment facility, for the physician to see their wives, for the results of the blood work, for the treatment to be over, and for prescriptions to be filled. Waiting was incessant, prolonged, boring, extremely irritating, anxiety provoking, and expected. Informants who accompanied their wives for admission to the hospital had to wait for the blood tests before they could be certain of admission. The informants experienced both the desire to return to work and the desire for the treatment to be completed, and this conflicting pressure made the hours of waiting seem longer.

Waiting was a time when "everything went through your mind, mostly about cancer. That was all you thought about." The lack of choice was frustrating: "You have to sit and wait your turn. What else can you do?" The informants wondered how women who came alone managed to wait without "someone to lean on." Several informants found the waiting particularly stressful because the physicians were uncommunicative. They waited hoping to hear something positive but they were never told anything.

The fight was measured by the results of diagnostic tests which were not routine but controlled by the physician. Uncertainty about when the tests were to be done or "how the tests are going to work out" influenced the waiting: "It was always the same every time. It was always hoping and praying that things are still going to work out." One couple had to wait 11 months before a CAT scan:

> Up until that point, we did not know whether there was any hope or not. It is in that period of time that people find themselves in total distress.

Anger at the system, the lack of compassion from health care providers, and the long wait for test results influenced the informants' coping strategies. They felt that being forced to wait up to five days to get test results showed a lack of compassion, and they found it demeaning when scans were not shown to them, particularly when the wife was using creative visualization (an alternative form of holistic healing) and needed to see the scans. Whether the informants phoned or personally requested information they were often unsuccessful.

Committing

Although all of the informants decided to help their wives endure the effects of chemotherapy treatments, the factors that influenced their decisions varied. Those who had been married a long time stayed to help because they considered their loyalty was fair. The informants knew they would not like to undergo chemotherapy treatment alone and they felt sorry for women who were alone. Other factors influencing the decision to help were moral values, guilt, the determination of the wives to fight, and the length of the chemotherapy treatment. In most case the resolution to fight, made when the threat was first identified, was firm and not negotiable. Factors that influenced a reevaluation included the promise of inheritance, previous successful chemotherapy, and a genuine compassion or love for their wives. Indecisiveness was influenced by frustration and anger with their wives' temperament, a belief the illness was not life-threatening, a new job, a lack of love for the wife, and a relationship with another woman.

The informants were aware of husbands who had separated from their wives, and they believed the reason for leaving was the increased stress in conjunction with an inability to respond positively to the wife's behavior. The uncertainty of the outcome of treatment along with the prolonged period of waiting associated with "not knowing what's going to happen" was indeterminable: "So I can see how easy it would be just to walk and say, see you later, you know, it's your problem."

Implementing Strategies

Informants began to plan and implement ways to buffer. When the informants' ability to implement strategies was compared with their ability to resolve anger, attitudes became obvious (see Figure 6.6).

Those informants who dissipated their anger maintained a positive attitude (Figure 6.6, Cell *a*). They were able to grow within the limitations imposed by the cancer experience and they accepted the need to participate. Husbands who expressed anger but were not able to implement strategies lacked self-control (Figure 6.6, Cell *b*). These informants often lacked emotions or were physically ill. Their concern was often focused on themselves and they showed a lack of concern for others. These informants were minimally involved in helping their wives. Husbands who were unable to express anger were often very stressed (Figure 6.6, Cell *c*). If employed, they spent an increasing amount of time at work. They usually accompanied their wives to treatment and never seemed able to do enough for their wives. These informants were always rushed, had high self-expectations, and did not like to discuss the cancer experience. The fourth cell describes informants who were unable either to express their anger or implement effective strategies, and these informants were bitter and negative (Figure 6.6, Cell *d*). They felt like failures because they received little positive feedback. They never spoke with anyone about the cancer experience and they withdrew when others wanted to share experiences with them.

The informants assisted their wives by softening the blow, resisting disruption, and preserving self. *Softening the blow* involved strategies that were supporting, endearing, and designed to make day-to-day life easier. *Resisting disruption* involved denying those

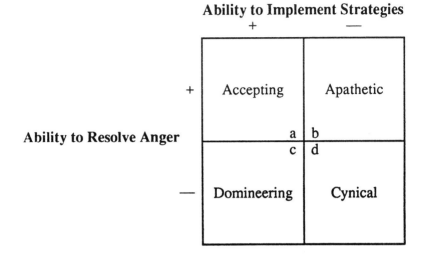

Figure 6.6. The Relationship Between the Husband's Ability to Resolve Anger and his Ability to Assist his Wife to Endure Chemotherapy

behaviors known to disrupt day-to-day life and preserving self-involved strategies the informants used to help themselves.

Softening the Blow

The informants provided supportive care: "You do whatever you have to for someone you love to make it as easy as possible. Everything I did was strictly for my wife. I had to do everything to make it easier." The philosophy was that "anybody who had cancer must also have a fear of death that was second to none." They believed that

> if you want to survive the situation, you really have to turn yourself into something that can be helpful to the person that's sick.

> You just can't go through that kind of experience by yourself. There's just too many things happening emotionally and physically. You need someone that is close to you.

Even when resisted by their wives the informants felt that effective caring had to be continuous, constant, and persistent. The informants in this study felt that being there, cherishing, normalizing, being positive, taking charge, and adding on were supportive measures.

Being there. Being there meant one had to be egotistical, had to believe in himself and the necessity of his role, and had to become an "insider" who knew and understood chemotherapy: "She wants me with her. I want to be there. It's a mutual thing." The cancer experience often isolated the couple and they had to support each other: "I go home with the anticipation of helping her cope. I know I have got to help." The cancer experience required the informants to assume different roles, for example one husband had to be a friend because his wife talked to no one else. *Being there* meant knowing enough to leave wives alone and not hover over them, restricting their independence. Some of the informants took early retirement or denied themselves enjoyable leisure activities. Often, *being there* was evaluated by the guilt the informants could expect to experience if they did something else.

Being there and getting ready for chemotherapy became routine. Informants "stocked up" on liquids or food their wives could tolerate. Sometimes conversation would dwell on the best site for chemotherapy injections, but usually the informants used distractions to "take the edge off the evening." In spite of their willingness to be there the informants always felt a secret, underlying sadness, which was never verbalized, when getting ready for treatment.

Experiences during chemotherapy differed according to the setting. One informant, who had visited and found his wife on life-support machines, looking "ready to die," was always afraid when he entered the hospital. Another informant witnessed an emergency in which the patient died, and after this incident he wanted to be constantly with his wife. Receiving treatment in an outpatient facility that offered small separate rooms had the advantage of privacy and this setting offered the informant the opportunity to stay with his wife. Unfortunately, these rooms were like "jail cells" after 14 months of chemotherapy. In most cases chemotherapy was given to everyone together in a small outpatient room, and the informants felt inadequate in their attempts to allay their wives' nervousness in the presence of others. Rarely did couples touch or talk to each other in any setting.

During chemotherapy infusion the informants were present when their wives requested their presence. Many of the informants felt "in the way" of the nurses due to the size of the room, availability of chairs to sit on, and the number of patients in the room. Some of the informants waited in the hallway until the needles were inserted for chemotherapy and then they entered the treatment room. The clinic was always busy and the informants worried that the other women would be resentful when their own husbands were not present. One informant saw women alone and crying after treatment, which reinforced his determination to be with his wife. Although crying was rarely seen, the informants observed signs of nervousness and anxiety in other patients. Although they wanted to be there, they became claustrophobic, bored, restless, and ached to leave. Often they would find excuses to leave, such as going to put money in the parking meter. Those who had been accompanying their wives for some time often recognized familiar faces.

Cherishing. Cherishing consisted of nurturing, listening, touching, humoring, and "doing" for wives. Informants changed, becoming more attentive, compassionate, and considerate. They wanted "to be able to do more," and they no longer took their wives "for granted." The emotions of affection, gratitude, and love expressed by the informants were similar to the "honeymoon stage" of newlyweds. The informants found solace in the marital relationship even though sexual activity had decreased. Although the "opportunities were always there to be unfaithful," and there was "no question about it, the thought sure enters your mind," most of the informants were loyal. Often, childhood experiences affected their faithfulness. One informant's mother had been abandoned by her husband leaving her with two small children, and he remembered what that had been like for his mother.

The informants most frequently considered their wives' basic needs for rest, sleep, and nutrition. For some touch took on healing powers as back rubs, neck rubs, and hugs were relaxing and comforting; however, some wives resisted any form of touch. In spite of feeling rejected the informants provided physical care such as bathing or homemaking tasks such as cooking. Work behavior changed and working overtime became nonexistent. When unable to be there, the informants asked friends or relatives to stay or they hired someone to care for their wives in the home.

Nurturing included caring, loving, and supporting their wives in order to make them "feel better," but the informants were careful not to overdo cheerfulness or "cheapen themselves." The informants knew too many compliments given unwisely would sound dishonest or "phoney." Wives were depressed and dissatisfied, causing them to question their husbands' love; therefore, how a compliment was given influenced the wife's self-image. Many of the informants believed they came to love their wives more deeply than before and wanted to convey this love. They tried not to be patronizing and learned not to say "I understand how you feel" because they knew no one could really understand unless they had experienced chemotherapy. Some informants spent a great deal of money "spoiling" their wives. The spoiling by spending money gave informants satisfaction and positive feedback because it was something to "give up" just as their wife was giving up a lot of her energy to undergo chemotherapy. For example, one informant said there was "nothing I won't do. If she wants something, I do it. Anything within my power, I'll do." Another informant was told by his wife that he was doing too much, and upon reflection he realized that at that time he was not listening nor could he have changed. Informants wanted "to make her well" and expressed "feeling lost." They hoped that what they were doing was enough, that it was "the right thing."

The informants believed that their wives needed to have someone nearby who loved them. Wives were more afraid of being abandoned and left alone than of their husbands having an extramarital affair. In order to reassure wives of their fidelity the informants were present in the home for longer periods. They rushed home from work and *being there* became important for maintaining trust in the relationship. Many of the informants telephoned their wives throughout the day just "to give her a chance to talk."

For some of the informants caring meant accepting changes and assuming passivity, such as following a new diet they did not like because it was important to their wives or accepting anger by ignoring caustic remarks. Humor "lightened things up a little bit" and reduced "tense situations," and it was "something to take her mind off her problems." Some of the wives lost their sense of humor, making it difficult to judge how and when to try "to be funny." A smile offered immediate feedback: "The best time I have, really, is when she laughs."

Wives wanted to discuss what they were reading, and they wanted someone to listen: "I learned to keep my mouth shut through sheer experience. I'd often just sit there and not say a word for two hours." Listening, a learned response, involved "sitting nearby and giving eye contact," but this was not comfortable for those informants used to action. Listening had two outcomes: it helped wives "vent some of their problems and get them out of the way," and the informants learned what their wives were thinking about.

Normalizing. Normalizing meant maintaining a life-style close to the way it was before the cancer experience. Informants tried to "do the same thing every day that I normally do" around home because routine was supportive in its familiarity. Although some of the informants said they were frustrated because they had to do everything, home maintenance was important: "You don't stop living because something has changed within the family unit." When children were living in the home tasks were often delegated. Informants believed "pitching in more" with these tasks "made things easier" for their wives. Weekly routines such as going to church were maintained even when the wives did not accompany the family.

The informants believed social interaction provided healthy distractions from the cancer experience, and getting out of the home made one feel less isolated and withdrawn and created "a little better outlook on life." The informants believed their wives needed to "get out once in a while" because they were alone so much, and they "needed a chance to enjoy life." Usually, social activities decreased because the wives were in bed earlier.

Children needed to be informed of their mother's illness. Older children were informed in greater detail than younger children. Informants, who usually told their children, would not discuss the extent of their wives' suffering. Telling a daughter that her mother might die was devastating for one informant, and even when he knew his wife was dying, he never told his daughter "exactly." Daughters cried and were not calm in their acceptance, although sons tended to be more stoic. Because of the concentration on the marital dyad older children were often ignored, although informants with younger children assumed "mothering tasks."

Taking charge. Taking charge usually involved isolated behaviors designed to protect the wives' well-being. *Taking charge* usurped the *doer* role in that the informant made quick judgments about the value of something and became totally committed. Anger was often the impetus for *taking charge* behavior, for example one informant telephoned the Minister of Health and "had a fight with him" because his comments in the newspaper reflected a lack of understanding about the cancer experience. Another informant controlled the television shows his wife saw so that she only watched those that had a "happy ending." *Taking charge* was often legitimized by a wife's request. For example, in spite of the physician's belief that his wife was dehydrated, needed fluid, and would not be discharged until the next day, one informant's wife requested that he "get [her] out of this hospital": "We checked out at midnight."

Informants worried about the "pills" their wives were expected to consume and they assumed the task of making certain their wives took the right pill at the right time, which was very difficult when the informants worked. One wife telephoned her husband crying because she had fallen asleep and missed a pill. In this instance, *taking charge* involved a series of actions used to identify which pill had been missed and what to do about it. Another informant said that during the appointment with the physician *taking charge* meant reminding his wife when she forgot to inform the physician about instances of duress. He knew the physician would then question the wife in more depth. When someone upset the wife, they were no longer welcome in their home. For example, one relative used to talk about "all the people who did not make it," and this relative was told by the informant not to visit or talk with his wife again.

Being positive. Being positive allowed the informants to hope even in the face of *guarded optimism* and to live one day at a time. *Being positive* was confidence-building, and it helped the informants temporarily repress their fear of the cancer experience. The informants thought that both spouses must be positive in order to be effective:

Do not let whatever is happening get to you so that you start feeling negative. Once you start feeling negative, then you have a problem. If it was both of you feeling negative, somebody else will have to come in and get you back on a positive note.

The informants said *being positive* was a source of support: "If I was positive about things and trying to make my wife positive, then she would feel better. In turn, I would feel better." *Being positive* was believed to affect the length of survival, and his attitude presumed that "the getting well process was within oneself" and not only in the realm of medicine.

The informants found it difficult to be positive when their wives experienced a recurrence of the disease or when a treatment had been cancelled. Often, *being positive* was the strategy used to "pull" wives out of a bad mood. When one spouse was not as positive as the other, they "hoped that it was never on the same day." To prevent this it was important to recognize what the other spouse was feeling and try not to be "down" at the same time. Therefore, this strategy meant that the couple had to trust each other and not keep secrets. The assumption was that keeping secrets from someone who knew the other so well was impossible because they would "pick that up right away." When one did have a secret, it was very stressful and guilt-producing. For example, one informant had been informed of his wife's survival time by the physician and the secret of knowing made him nervous about his wife's potential resentment.

The informants said *being positive* in the face of dismal statistics was difficult, so they either considered them meaningless or denied them: "We will not be one of those statistics." The informants' fear increased when physicians did not offer any guarantee or positive encouragement to the couple; consequently, the informants often looked to nurses as a source of hope, but they felt the nurses "didn't want to be responsible for throwing out a ray of hope." As a result, the informants learned to follow "orders" and not to ask questions because they really did not want to find out something that would make them "more negative, or more uncertain."

Being positive meant finding reasons to be hopeful, such as seeking out information about successes with chemotherapy. Talking with someone who had finished their chemotherapy and could get "back to their normal life" inspired hope. Hope was enriched when their wives felt better, believed they were going to get better, or went into remission. One informant believed hope was conditional, but *being positive* left no room for doubt. Although one informant felt not making long-term goals implied being less hopeful, *being positive* usually meant making reachable short-term goals. Praying or going to church helped some of the informants stay positive because it helped them accentuate the positive things about living. Comparing oneself to others made the informants feel lucky, and some of them "soaked up" all their friends' and relatives' "positive vibes" in order to enhance hopefulness.

The informants said the process of maintaining a positive attitude depleted their energy. One informant described the process of *being positive* as self-teaching or brainwashing. *Being positive* involved "self-control and not letting the mind get out of control." Self-control involved knowing the self well enough to be able to control negative feelings. For some it took "double the effort" because they had to be positive for themselves as well as for their wives. Those informants whose wives died said they had always hoped something "might turn up" to help their wives. These informants felt that as long as they could implement strategies to help themselves remain positive they could influence their wives' attitude. One of the worst dilemmas for the informants in this study was when they could not be hopeful and could not honestly maintain a positive attitude.

Adding on. Adding on was being innovative, trying alternative means to augment the conventional treatment of chemotherapy. *Adding on* allowed the couple to experiment with their treatment and it gave them some measure of choice and control. *Adding on* was believed to increase the chances of a better outcome of treatment. Often, the emphasis was on practicing those alternative methods chosen by the couple and simultaneously "putting them all together" so they could act as catalysts for each other.

Reading everything they could get their hands on and discussing approaches with the nurse or physician encouraged innovations. Methods included creative visualization and imagery, dietary regimens, relaxation therapy, prayer and the belief that one can heal oneself with God's help, cessation of smoking, increasing contributions to the cancer society, exercise (such as yoga) meditation, seeking counseling services, submitting to healing ceremonies, and wearing a magnet or grounding stone.

Resisting Disruption

The wives experienced periods of boredom and were vulnerable. The informants were never sure when their wives would be bored and they felt they had to maintain self-control at all times in order to be helpful. They believed their wives' attitudes of determination and optimism helped make the cancer experience easier for themselves; consequently the informants felt that in order to repay their wives they had to resist disruption in order to enhance normalization. One informant said that he

> tried everything in his power not to cry or show any emotion towards her disease or her condition, to go on with life as if nothing happened. But deep down, you know you are doing it for a reason.

The informants wanted to be the closest person to their wives and they did this by disguising their feelings: "I did what I thought was best for her, what was right, at the time." The informants had to decide for themselves what this "right" thing was because talking to other husbands in similar situations was rare.

Disguising one's feelings. The informants thought their anger or doubt would impede their wives' ability to fight, and they felt they had to be devious in disguising these emotions: "She would pick that up right away. That is one of the things that scares me." One of the informants said he "felt he was wearing a mask," and it was "very stressful being somebody that he was not."

Many of the informants believed that talking about their own feelings threatened their self-control: "I tried to do a good job of hiding my feelings from her. I never wanted to show weakness in front of her." The informants felt crying in front of their wives was unforgivable because it indicated a lack of self-control. One informant said he "did break down and she was really worried"; while another informant felt his wife was "just barely hanging on to her sanity," and he was sure his crying would push her toward insanity. Some of the informants felt crying represented "feeling sorry for yourself." Losing control, becoming impatient, and, above all, being patronizing, condescending, or intrusive were behaviors avoided by the informants in this study.

The informants never considered sharing their feelings with their wives: "I did not think I could ever unload that on her." The informants said it was easier to talk about these feelings "after she was gone" than while she was alive, and many of the informants could not "remember ever telling their wives how they felt about it [the cancer experience]." Even though the informants did not express their feelings to their wives, most of them wanted to talk to someone about their feelings: "I wanted to tell somebody. How does somebody get that feeling out of their stomach, of watching someone you love going through chemotherapy?" Several tried to talk to their wives about their feelings, but they found that their wives did not want to listen. For example, one wife told her husband to "shut up."

The informants said they never discussed their feelings of *guarded optimism* with their wives. When hearing of a good test result, the informants were hesitant to become ecstatic "because you were not sure if it was real or not." They hoped the test result was real, but they were afraid to be optimistic: "You can only put yourself [through] so many ups and downs."

Treading lightly. Treading lightly was a strategy the informants used to avoid unpleasantness. When *treading lightly* the informants assumed a passive, supporter role. The informants said that *treading lightly* involved not saying "the wrong thing" or expressing something in "the wrong way." The wrong way was learned through experience and "trial and error." They had to be very careful because once something was said or done it could not be undone. One informant said he had expressed a concern over finances when his wife was seeing a psychologist. After six visits, he had asked his wife if she felt better after talking with the psychologist. She quickly asked why, without commenting on his enquiry. He did not have time to formulate an answer and instinctively showed her the bill for services, which made him feel guilty for bringing it up instead of just paying the bill. After this incident, his wife would not consider going back to the psychologist or finding another person who might be less expensive; in fact, this wife resisted all of her husband's attempts to change her mind. The incident was devastating for him because he was afraid he had impeded her ability to cope with the chemotherapy experience.

Many of the informants became so distrustful of their own ability to respond they were almost afraid to talk to their wives. Solutions included becoming "listeners," waiting until their wives talked to them, not "trying to start a conversation," avoiding the "wrongs" by doing more "rights," and hoping for the best. Although the informants were trying to maintain a normal life-style they were aware of things they should or should not do. The informants felt as though they were walking a tightrope, trying to create a life-style with balance so that neither spouse became upset or anxious and every emotional crisis was averted. One informant described treading lightly as "walking on eggshells."

Anger created a dilemma for the informants. Some of them said they would leave rather than argue, and although in a "slightly milder" way others acted normally and "snapped back." The dilemma for the informants existed in their desire for a normal life and their desire to make their wives feel less like invalids. Although they wanted to "let her know that there wasn't any cause to speak to me that way," they also wanted to avoid an argument. For many of the informants, the diplomatic approach was difficult.

Treading lightly allowed the informants to perform the *doer* role, which helped their own self-esteem. They felt they could not allow a role reversal, that is, wives comforting or pleasing them: "I did not want her comforting me, that would be bad." Above all they did not want their wives feeling helpless, and they thought their wives should feel free to be selfish.

The one topic informants were uncertain about discussing was sexual activity. They said they felt unsure about how to engage in sexual activity, and although some couples resumed sexual activities it was usually not to the degree they had enjoyed before the cancer experience. Those informants who did not resume sexual relations believed their wives felt sexually inadequate due to the changes brought about by the surgery or chemotherapy. Some wives experienced pain during intercourse, and others felt neutered and unattractive. Because the informants did not want their wives to interpret the lack of sexual intimacy as a reflection of their love, they were placed in a dilemma. Some of the informants said they had to be careful not to communicate any romantic behaviors because their wives might interpret this as a sexual innuendo and find it threatening or frightening. Although some couples talked about their abstinence openly, most found it difficult to discuss their lack of sexual intimacy.

Discussing sexual relations was painful for the informant because the sexual response was part of their identity in the marital unit and it became more difficult if the couple did not usually share personal feelings with one another. The informants believed taking the path of least resistance relieved their wives of any undue stress; consequently, they did not discuss sexual relations.

Omitting the truth. Omitting the truth was a strategy used when the informants could not say something positive or complimentary, and they evaluated everything in terms of whether or not it was controversial. For example, they could not tell their wives they were looking great when they looked ill so they would say nothing. *Omitting the truth* included changing the subject or redirecting the discussion away from the wife's appearance. *Omitting the truth* was a defensive behavior; for example, the informants did not inform their wives about their increased drinking or smoking habits or about having a relationship with another woman. The informants felt this strategy was justified because it protected their wives from more suffering and it allowed the informants to continue supporting their wives even though they felt guilty.

Preserving self. The informants in this study became "self-supporters." A self-supporter conserves energy, maintains motivation, and sharpens his helping skills.

Conserving energy. Self-control was an important influence on the informants' behavior. For many, the need for self-control was uppermost in their minds:

> You police your own thinking. You have to be your own policeman. When you don't want to think about something, that's when you have to turn it off.

Through *conserving energy* and releasing tension the informants were able to maintain self-control. For some of the informants self-control culminated in positive thinking and affected how they projected themselves. A strategy for maintaining self-control was to find a way to release the accumulated tension. One informant had a "switch" he was able to turn off and on that helped him concentrate on his work during work hours and concentrate on helping his wife when at home. The switch helped him "block everything else out." Many of the informants released tension by finding a private place to yell, scream, or cry: "It is amazing at how the energy and tension flows out of you. That is part of the health of being able to do that. You heal yourself." For another, self-control meant controlling his own mind, and he used meditation, self-hypnosis, or yoga to change his state of mind.

Keeping busy. Keeping busy was one way the informants were able to focus their thoughts on something other than the chemotherapy experience. The wives who stated or inferred their desire to be alone gave their husbands permission to take care of themselves, and some of them were "happy to get out" on their own because going to and from work was the only private time they had for introspection and the expression of sadness.

Work, the most common way of *keeping busy,* was an escape from the informants' helpless situation. Work offered the informants the chance to be totally immersed in something other than their wives' cancer experience and they "didn't have much time to think about their own problems." For one informant, who communicated very little with his wife, work represented the "peace or companionship" not available at home. Work provided a different milieu with different things to think about. Work was like "stepping into another world," but as soon as the informants left work and got in their car to go home, the real world of the cancer experience was back. Retirement was not an alternative for most of the informants in this study and work was a legitimate part of their time away from home. Although working was a necessity, many felt guilty being away from their wives. For example, even though he needed the money gained by working, one informant felt guilty about "pushing his wife away when he went to work."

Several employers did not accommodate the informants needs and work became an intense stressor, producing a lot of anger. Two informants changed employment, two took early retirement, and another was ready to quit his job during this study. Many of the informants remained at work because of seniority, age, the need for income, or because they felt they had no choice. Others had flexibility in their work hours and colleagues who helped them when they needed it.

Healthiness. Exercise in the form of group sports (such as hockey) or individual sports (such as, running, swimming, or t'ai chi) was relaxing as it "helped to get rid of frustrations." Active sports kept the informants' energy level "up" during the day, and it helped them sleep through the night. Exercise was self-indulgent and it allowed the informants time to think. For some of the informants the enjoyment gained from exercising was undermined by guilt caused by the realization that they were enjoying something that their wives could not enjoy. Most of them resolved this dilemma by reasoning that their ability to support their wives often depended on energizing themselves through exercise. Most of them wanted to be feeling "the best I can if I am going to be of any use. I cannot afford to get sick." They took care of themselves with a proper diet, by getting enough sleep, and by getting enough exercise. Although many of them had periods of indulging early in the cancer experience, all of the informants became more aware of the need to look after themselves so that they could be useful to their wives.

Seeking other people. Seeking other people to talk to gave the informants a sense of personal satisfaction. Talking was doing something to help find meaning in the cancer experience, and it was described as "sharing your burden." Through sharing the informants came to understand more about the cancer experience and were able to formulate questions, which also helped them understand their wives' cancer experience. Some informants talked with physicians, nurses, priests, mothers, mothers-in-law, and friends, and most of them sought a male rather than a female to talk "at." Talking at required a good listener; whereas, talking "with" required a listener and a talker. Talking at let the informants "lay out their emotions, their feelings," and talking was particularly useful when they felt angry or down. The attributes of someone chosen to talk at were that he was caring, loving, compassionate, and knowledgeable about what informants were going through, and a good listener was someone who did not interrupt or question the informant.

It often took the wife's prodding to make the informant realize that he should seek help. The prodding freed him to talk with someone else because he was not betraying his wife's trust. Often, *seeking other people* involved talking with someone the informant had not known before, and this allowed him to express feelings that he could not verbalize to someone he knew. Talking with a stranger also "allowed the stream of consciousness to go" without making the informants feel like they were "laying a trip" on a friend; however, most informants did not want to talk or were not ready to talk and they admitted that even if someone had approached them they might not have talked. Others stated that it would have been better for them if they had found someone to talk to (for example, "an outsider" who was not sharing the experience with them personally) and they also said they would have appreciated "a little bit of prompting." Above all, the informants said they had to trust and like the person before they could talk about their experience of their wives' cancer experience.

One institution offered a meeting for husbands held one morning a week which was led by a clergyman. In order for husbands to avail themselves of this opportunity, treatment had to fall on that specific day. One husband found the group to be like a drop-in center, and although he was welcomed and talked with another husband he did not feel this was helpful for himself. He had not known what he expected to find helpful but he knew that he did not find it there.

Talking was considered acceptable when the focus remained on the wife. One informant, who described himself as tense and para-lyzed with fear during the whole time of his wife's illness, never talked openly with someone. His bitterness and anger endured and he wanted everyone "to stay away from him" because the last thing he wanted was "sympathy" or "anybody feeling sorry for me." For this informant talking meant being the recipient of sympathy, which might in turn make him feel sorry for himself. In the past he had "always talked with his wife" and "was not used to talking with a stranger." He admitted to feeling "not right" about going to talk with someone because he felt he would be divulging secrets or being weak. His question "Who was I going to talk to?" implied he really did not know where to turn at that time: "My mind was so screwed up anyway, but to try and straighten it out, it would have been definitely too much." He did have one good experience when a nurse approached him and talked with him; however, following their talk he felt he had said too much. As a result he felt weak for having talked to someone about his difficulties, and he wanted to apologize to the nurse but he never saw her again. In contrast, another inform-ant felt the need to talk about the cancer experience right from the beginning. He said he "could not pretend that nothing was happen-ing," and talking about it meant he was not denying his wife's illness.

He told his boss, which relieved him of trying to "hide" the knowledge from others. Telling his boss also enabled him to feel some flexibility and security at work, that is if his wife needed him and he had to leave work urgently his boss would understand.

Although most of the informants adhered to a code of secrecy established to curtail their own self-interest, one informant found talking helped him deal with his wife's rejection. He felt lonely and said that "bringing everything out in the open" was "mentally healthy." He felt he was going "stir crazy" staying in the home as his wife withdrew from any interaction. His intention to seek professional counseling indicated his need to remain normal and sane. The perceptions of others were also important to the informants. They thought they were coping, but when others told them what they were doing they were surprised. Receiving feedback from others was important to the informants for gaining insight into ways for conserving and channeling energy.

Maintaining motivation. The informants in this study appreciated compassionate and supportive friends: They knew "you were hurting" and "they did little things" to show they cared. This caring nurtured the informants and as a result they were able to nurture their wives. The informants also said they needed to be acknowledged in order to maintain their self-esteem and they rarely said "no" to any request from family members. The best motivator was their ability to say "I am doing the best that I can." When the informant could say this, he did not feel guilty about anything and was able to protect his self-esteem. Looking for feedback from physicians was ongoing because the informants felt they received little information from their wives' physicians. When physicians "looked pleased" or said, "She'll be all right," the informants were ecstatic.

One informant described himself as being in a "social worker role" when he talked with other husbands. By giving them hope he reinforced his own determination to be hopeful, but he found helping others did not help his positive attitude because they were always discussing someone else's problems and not his own. He wanted to be the one to motivate others but he found it difficult to ask others for help because he was considered an "expert" after years of experiencing his wife's chemotherapy. Consequently, he felt he should know how to help himself. These high expectations were also reflected in what he expected from physicians and nurses and he felt

constantly frustrated because he believed they were constantly failing him.

Knowing "that more people are surviving" chemotherapy and
seeing people who "have conquered this problem" helped supply
legitimate and inspiring proof of success. One informant said it made
a difference when he moved physically closer to his nuclear family
after chemotherapy. For some knowing statistics helped, but for
others the statistics were dismal and not helpful. Knowing those who
administered treatments, becoming familiar "with the place and the
people here," and normalizing the chemotherapy maintained the
informants' motivation to help their wives. Also, the informants felt
ignored by the nurses and they were not considered particularly
helpful. Rationalizing that nurses were there to spend time with their
wives did not make it any easier for the informants to accept being
ignored by the nursing staff.

Sharpening helping skills. By controlling their anger the informants sharpened their helping skills. Once anger was identified it
could be controlled, but many of the informants were unwilling to
acknowledge and express their anger. They were angry at the "torture" imposed by the chemotherapy and at the life-style changes
forced on them:

> I was mad, I was damn mad. I was mad at life. I was mad at everything. I
> had to give up my job. I had to do all these things I didn't want to do.

As one informant said, "Anger is something you don't want to repress
[because] you can become really disgusted with yourself." When
unable to express anger, the informants had to "try very hard not to
get angry at their wives," which created more stress. Anger was
described as "bad," "negative thinking," "stressful," and a "killer" that
one had to be careful of because it has "a sort of bitterness about it."
Anger was also associated with helplessness: "You can't do anything
about." Conversely, the release of anger was relaxing and rewarding.
Most of the informants felt they never got rid of all their anger;
however, they learned to control it through self-control.

The informants always tried to determine the effectiveness of a
particular helping strategy. They watched for signs of satisfaction
(such as when their wives smiled or were a little more "cheery") or
for tenseness (such as body posture and facial expressions). Some-

times the informants received feedback from a third party, for example, when a mother-in-law said that her daughter felt she was "very lucky" to have such an attentive husband. A smile was worth everything to the informants because it made them feel "that it was worth it." Being appreciated was considered "one of the benefits," and when a wife said, "Did I ever tell you I love you" or "I feel so safe when you are around me," the informant knew he was doing the right thing.

Helping inappropriately, such as when informants became too protective, made the wives feel dependent. Overprotectiveness was evident when the informants had difficulty leaving their wives alone. Many of them invented ways of ensuring their wives would be all right in their absence: For example, one informant would write down the times when his wife's pills were due and then would phone her from work to make certain she took them. Another informant did all the cooking and cleaning so that nothing was left for his wife to do when she was alone. Another had a friend come and stay with his wife when she was alone. This became a problem for some of the informants because they felt guilty when they realized their wives' had become dependent.

Finalizing

There were two specific emotive responses during the finalizing phase: relief and despair. The informants were relieved their wives "made it" and were finished with the chemotherapy treatments. Many of them did not initially talk about their relief; however, after a while, they learned to talk about it because "time has healed the wound." The informants did not have to identify themselves as the healthy ones any longer because they felt their wives were better. Time allowed the informants to "calm down," and they were relieved at no longer having to live by the calendar.

The informants felt the need to find something good in the experience and many of them believed the experience strengthened the family unit and the marital dyad. Others saw the experience "as a bit of an omen" which made them realize "life was a gift." Many of them felt they were being given the chance to change their life-style, and they were going to take advantage of the opportunity. Some of the informants began to put their wives "on a pedestal" as "you did not really appreciate her 'til you almost lose her."

For several informants the end of treatment meant despair because the chemotherapy was no longer effective in fighting the cancer. In most cases the chemotherapy was stopped by the physician, leaving the informant or his wife with no control over the decision to stop the chemotherapy treatments. When the couple was involved in the decision to stop chemotherapy they found it easier to accept the end of the treatments. One informant questioned the value of the treatment with the physician, and he was told it *might* prolong his wife's life for a few days. This informant did not want his wife to suffer needlessly, and he considered her quality of life before death. He discussed the efficacy of the treatment with her and then left the decision to her. She chose to stop the treatments and return home, which was a relief for both of them. In another case the wife stopped her treatments saying, "[I] would rather die than go through this, that this [is] absolutely no way to live. Living [is] good, but this [is] horrible." This wife had been enduring intermittent chemotherapy for six years with a cancer that progressed insidiously. Her husband said, "I was as relieved as she was when she decided no. We had discussed it, and she was prepared to die."

Several informants wondered if "life ever [got] back to normal?" as they continued waiting for tests. One informant described himself as optimistic but not eager for more chemotherapy. He felt it would be "as bad as the first time all over again." *Guarded optimism* surfaced as the informants hoped to "maintain this holding pattern." Part of the problem for many of the informants was that they could not see "an end in sight." They saw themselves waiting forever for test results and they felt it was "always going to be a little traumatic" waiting for test results. Trying to be realistic, one informant saw his wife returning for future "shots of chemo" until "they find a better way of dealing with it." Many of the informants felt "chemotherapy was better than death," and as long as their wives were being given treatment, the cancer was being treated and death was being denied.

Becoming a Veteran

The informants emerged from their wives' last administration of chemotherapy with a sense of fulfillment. They recognized the changes brought about by the chemotherapy, and they had a new perspective on the nature of waiting or marking time. Figure 6.7 depicts this process.

Making It Through

Being a veteran of the chemotherapy experience had lasting effects because of the unforgettable memory of such a devastating experience. Although their wives had made it through the informants could not forget that cancer can be deadly; and as a result they reverted back to "the waiting game. . . . Is it going to develop in another part of her body?" Once again they began to hope that the cancer experience was behind them: "We hope we do not have to repeat it again." Some of the informants celebrated reaching "the top of the mountain" by doing something pleasurable, for example taking a holiday with their wives.

All of the informants expressed pride and admiration for their wives' endurance during the chemotherapy treatments: "I think that is just incredible, to go through that horrendous experience and still come out with a sense of humor." They were in awe of their wives' ability to endure the experience and they wondered if they would have endured as well.

After the chemotherapy was finished, waiting to find out if the fight had been successful was a stressful time for the informants. The first check-up and set of diagnostic tests would be the best indicator and the couples waited anxiously for the results of these tests. Although some of the couples continued to talk of "cure," many considered the words "control" and "remission" to be more applicable to their fight: "A lot of people think that a cancer, once cured, cannot return, but a cancer can return as it is within the system." Although this man's wife had not experienced a recurrence his remarks reflect the *guarded optimism* that was always present.

The informants had learned to accept "the thing," and now, they wanted to "have fun" because they had made it through the experience. It was time to get on with living "some sort of normal way of life." The informants felt they had done the "best that we could so far," and this attitude indicated that although it was not over yet they were "trying to be optimistic." Some of the informants wanted to "repay the favor" by doing something for others who were not as fortunate. One young couple had endured "heavy" chemotherapy

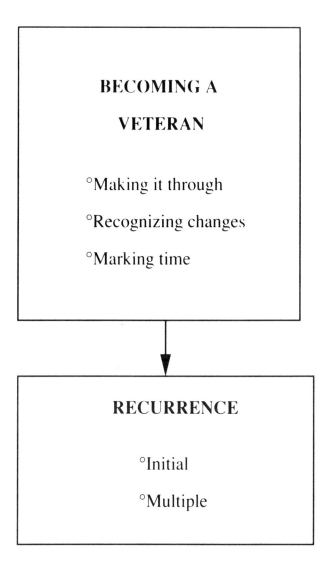

Figure 6.7. The Process of Emerging as a Veteran

for three months, and they considered themselves lucky they were able to "get it over with quickly." They began to think of getting involved with helping others almost immediately after completing their own course of treatment.

At the completion of chemotherapy treatments the informants evaluated and assessed the things they would change in their lives. Changes included not interfering with their wives' life-style and not letting their own day-to-day life revolve around the *doer* role to the exclusion of everything else. As a result, they were left with more time and energy. One informant became so involved in his role that afterward he said, "Maybe I'm lost, maybe I got lost as a result of this devastation. I don't know what the heck to do with myself now."

Stress increased as the couple approached check-up times and the informants said it was hard to relax until after the first check-up. The worry about a recurrence was something that some of the informants adapted to, although others could not "relax until about five years from now. If you can make it to five years, you have probably had the problems cured." The "magic five-year point" was a common belief in the *making it through* phase, and the informants continued watching the calendar. Although chemotherapy was "a means to an end," the uncertainty of "how it is all going to turn out" was now the "hardest part, without a doubt."

Recognizing Changes

Guarded optimism reappeared as the informants wondered if their wives would ever return to their "old selves," to the way they were before the chemotherapy treatments. The informants believed thoughts of "normalcy" were idealistic, and they wondered if they were "just fooling themselves." In spite of their *guarded optimism* the informants recognized changes in their wives. Wives were not as self-centered: "We are not *I* anymore. We are *we,* and we are together." At this time the informants decided "things were going to be okay." The biggest physical change noticed by the informants was the growth of fine hair. One husband described this event as the "real turning point" for his wife. Although wives continued to need a lot of sleep, skin color improved daily, and their strength and stamina began to improve as they began to engage in more activities.

The most significant changes for the informants were the emotional ones: "She was more like she used to be." The regrowth of hair was considered to be the greatest factor contributing to the stabilization of the wives' moods. Several informants described their wives as "a different woman" who was more outgoing, began participating in different activities, and started to "come out of that shell she was in." The physicians warned that unexplainable social, emotional, or physical changes could occur as a result of the chemotherapy, and the informants were constantly vigilant for these unexplainable changes. Changes were noted for up to two years after the wife had finished her chemotherapy treatment. A change in memory and slowed mental processes were noted by all of the informants.

Many of the informants experienced residual anger. They were angry at "things" or "others" rather than themselves, their wives, or the nurses. Sometimes anger was directed toward the physician or a particular situation, for example having to move in order to be closer to the family or the treatment facility. Of those informants whose wives died, many were still angry "at what happened," and they missed their wives. One informant left the Roman Catholic church because he could not understand how a loving God could do such a thing to his wife. He did not want to get involved with the people at the church anymore. Although many of the informants in this study became "very upset, very emotional" when reliving the experience, all of them felt talking about their wives' chemotherapy had been a positive experience.

The informants also described changes in themselves. These changes were attributed to their belief that their wives were "getting well." Changes included a greater freedom to enjoy life, using a physician for personal health concerns more frequently and having more patience and tolerance. The informants also experienced some emotional changes, particularly in the way they looked at the world around them. Comments ranged from "it made a new man out of me" to "everything was totally different." One informant described seeing other husbands change as he watched them during his wife's illness. He noted changes in the way they talked with other people, and he saw everyone go through a stage of feeling sorry for themselves. He believed that everyone went through the recurring stage of "feeling sorry for himself" and that some times were worse than others. He said that the experience either made husbands more sensitive, "more in tune with other people's feelings, more open-minded," or it made them "extremely hard, bitter, and insensitive to other's feelings." He contended that the husband who went through the experience with his wife had so much going on around him, "so much emotion, so much action, so much happening," that he had to change in response.

Many of the strategies the informants learned became entrenched in their personal coping repertoire; for example, bitterness continued for one informant. He said he could probably change his attitude but it would take more effort than he was willing to expend. Some of the informants said the cancer experience had caused them to age and/or alter their career goals. The informants also said the nightmares they experienced during the chemotherapy began to subside.

Most of the informants continued to live day-to-day, and they adhered to the philosophy that something good came from going through adversity. They believed the experience made them better men: "It was an interesting experience. You would like everybody to go through it and gain the experience but not to have the emotional upset." Many of the informants realized their life-style had been one in which they had taken too much for granted, and they vowed to change. Others recognized they had learned "not to say the wrong thing"; whereas before the experience they would have said whatever was on their minds. Other informants found they were now able to "sit and listen to people, and feel their feelings" with more insight and sensitivity, and many of them experienced the freedom to dream and make long-term plans: "We are making plans for the new year, and it is nice to look ahead again."

Marking Time

For the informants in this study, waiting (or *marking time*) was looking for the unexpected and never knowing if the cancer was going to recur. The informants were thankful when the treatments were over and hopeful of a cure, but they were afraid to be too optimistic, believing that attitude might be denying reality. As time passed, good check-ups were tallied and this fear decreased.

With no more chemotherapy to plan the days around, life got back to "normal." Wives often went back to work and were able to manage homemaking. The couple could now spend their money on things they enjoyed doing and holidays and trips became frequent. They also began to socialize more and they did not feel the need to isolate themselves from friends. The informants found they were now able to "talk freely and openly about the situation, without fear of breaking down." The informants became more confident as check-ups passed with no evidence of cancer. Memories of the horror faded and the informants began setting long-term goals so that their wives could look forward to pleasant things.

During this time, however, waiting was stressful because without treatments there was nothing to fight the cancer if it was growing. The first few check-ups supplied a sense of security as the wife was given indicators that her chemotherapy treatments had been successful. The periods between check-ups were silent and uneventful unless the wife developed symptoms. Diagnostic tests (such as scans) were done at the time of check-ups, which were usually conducted at three-month intervals after cessation of the chemotherapy. This time often seemed very long to the couple, and it was very difficult to keep hoping when they were wondering "Is it getting better?"

Sometimes the informants were unable to protect their wives. One wife went for a job interview and had to identify her health status and health history. The employer asked about her probability for survival. Another informant encountered a problem when applying for a loan. The loan was denied because of the possible loss of the wife's earning power if the cancer recurred. Also, life insurance was often denied.

For the informants the fear of recurrence "crept into their thoughts every so often"; but when this was weighed against having come through the chemotherapy and the fact that their wives looked well, the informants were usually able to repress these thoughts with less and less effort. Thoughts such as "the feeling that I might have to go through that again someday" were kept secret. It was more difficult for the informants to repress these thoughts when they knew someone who had experienced a recurrence of cancer or who had died from cancer: "There are always those fears in the back of your mind, that things are not going to be the way you really want." When wives worried, the informants worried.

The informants did not want to "dredge it up and go through the pain they had already gone through"; however, when with an insider they were more empathetic and caring. An insider was someone who was a survivor or who lived with someone who had cancer, and an outsider was someone who had no idea about the disease or the experiences of people who live with it:

> I really care for the insider who has to live with someone who has the disease. I really feel for them because I know exactly what they are going through. I try to give them help and encouragement.

The informants felt they had done everything they could do and "thanked God their wife had not had anything show up." Many of them believed that this was their "acceptance stage": That is, once the fight was over, they could look back and accept it, something they could not do while going through the fight. Although the informants were euphoric during this period, their wives often commented on death and dying: "I might not be here next year." These types of comments were difficult for the informants because they "were not sure how to react."

When considering the possibility of recurrence all of the informants said it would be worth going through chemotherapy again because it would mean prolonging their wives' lives. Although they did not want to consider the "what if," they were sure their wives would also choose to undergo chemotherapy again:

> I know that my wife would not want to go through it again. She did not like going through it the first time, but if it's a necessary evil, then I suppose that she would go through it.

The informants did not plan for a recurrence: "We will have to deal with that particular conflict at that time." Instead, they were more concerned with test results than with observing their wives for visible body changes.

Some of the informants become political advocates for cancer patients. Strategies included writing letters to Members of Parliament, campaigning for funds, campaigning for a better facility, and writing letters to the institution suggesting ways for improving care. One informant, who could not go near the clinic without feeling physically ill, campaigned for the Cancer Society. Interest in anything to do with cancer grew as the informants continued to read current news and media releases about the disease. Parents considered the risk to their children and practiced prevention (for example, making sure their children went to a reliable physician for check-ups and by teaching children self-examination principles) because "you just hope you do not get it. I would be devastated if my children got cancer."

For those informants whose wives had withdrawn from chemotherapy or who had the treatment stopped by the physician, there was "no wonderment anymore" because the couples knew why chemotherapy was stopped. One informant felt happy to be the one looking after his wife in the home: "You are there, and you can do everything that has to be done right now." He wanted to be with his wife without hospital personnel around interrupting their closeness, and it was easier for their friends to visit in the comfortable atmosphere of their home. At this point in the treatment the informants believed their wives had already accepted the fact that their disease was leading to death and that the point of dying was "not far off."

Recurrence

The recurrence of cancer in some other part of the body recycled the informants back into the process of identifying the threat, engaging in the fight, and becoming a veteran.

Initial Recurrence

After chemotherapy treatment, waiting for the three month checkup and for an indication of the success or failure of the treatment was stressful for the informants in this study. They began wondering whether the cancer was spreading and they often imagined that it was spreading. They looked for signs of disease progression, and they considered the difference between curing and controlling the disease. Controlling the disease was stopping the growth or progression of the cancer without completely curing or eradicating it. Metastases, or the spreading of cancer within the body, was feared, especially if it spread to the bone, liver, or pancreas. For the informants, recurrence meant the disease was winning, death was inevitable, and "the days were numbered."

Any amount of waiting became even more difficult once the cancer started spreading:

It seemed as if you were getting back on that old treadmill again. Now you know what it is. Your hopes were not is it or isn't it spreading, but rather, is it or isn't it getting better or worse? You were always hoping that there was some sign of remission or some sign that something was working.

When waiting for test results the couples sat quietly and did not talk about remission. Test results were awaited impatiently because they were a measure of disease progression and something upon which the informants based their hope. During this period the time spent waiting was worse than any other time because now the informants could not adapt to anything concrete, such as surgery or chemotherapy. One informant said the "big five-year obstacle" was almost insurmountable, and he was "very uptight all the time" because it was something he had to think about and plan for constantly. For another informant, finding out meant waiting because he had been informed by the physician that his wife's death was imminent. She lived much longer than expected and all he could do was wait patiently while trying to be supportive. In this case, the informant had trusted the physician's prognosis, and as a result he had to try to deal with the guilt associated with presumptuously preparing for his wife's death.

Even when the three month check-up had passed the informants continued *suspecting* behaviors. Some wives found abnormalities and the informants began to worry in earnest. One informant, whose wife found a breast lump, "prepared for the worst" only to have "it turn out well." Other informants reassured their wives, telling them to go back to physicians they trusted. One informant, whose wife found "lumps on her neck," examined these lumps, became worried, and acted. This couple went to the physician, who offered medication for stress headaches, implying the symptoms were the wife's fault and not due to a progression of disease. Although the physician did not positively diagnose their suspicions he did suggest more chemotherapy. In this case, *finding out* was very subtle, and it was difficult for the informant to *face the fact*. In other cases, the informants experienced existential concerns about death. These concerns were often due to the increased knowledge acquired during the chemotherapy process; for example, they learned that metastases always occurs prior to death.

One informant became anxious when his wife began acting out following unexpected news from her physician. His wife isolated

herself more than before and withdrew into her own world, and this
informant tried to *second-guess* her responses in order to understand
her. This informant worried about a missed treatment, its affect on
the disease progression, his responses to his wife's moods, and how
he could implement strategies to cope with recurrence. His strategies
included *preserving self* and changing his life-style and his relationships with others. Although this informant had no doubt his wife
would accept treatment, she had not decided whether she would
return for chemotherapy. He felt his wife's anger toward the cancer
was being placed on the physician, and he tried to implement
strategies that would ensure her decision for further chemotherapy.

Sometimes the first exposure to chemotherapy was as a treatment
for recurrence. One informant described the "process of emotional
letdown" he experienced during the chemotherapy. He felt the worst
part of the cancer experience, which lasted six years, was the struggle with suffering, even though the chemotherapy prolonged his
wife's life for another year.

Remission, or cessation of the cancer progression, was a great
relief: "It felt as if a great burden had been lifted off of our shoulders."
Another informant described remission as being as good as a cure.
Living with uncertainty and waiting became integrated in day-to-day
living, and looking to others for inspiration took on new meaning as
the informants became hopeful about controlling the disease.

Multiple Recurrence

Being informed by telephone was helpful for those informants
who found out about a recurrence of the cancer. The underlying
assumption was that the informant would tell his wife about the
extent of her disease; and for one informant this approach allowed
him time to express his disappointment privately before telling his
wife, and he felt better prepared "to handle it." He felt he could tell
his wife in a more humane manner than the physician because he
could tell her when, where, and how he wanted, and this allowed
him to maintain control of the situation.

Even though the "ring of familiarity sounded [on being informed],"
the informants still felt devastated. Although informants felt better
equipped knowing what to expect and what to do, they still experienced shock and fear. Some of the informants said they were better
equipped to deal with a recurrence because they had not gone

directly from surgery to chemotherapy, although others said they accepted the disease more readily because they had been through the fight before and lived with it longer. Even so, the informants were never completely prepared because the experience was never the same.

Witnessing a couple whose cancer had returned was difficult for the informants, and it made them realize that remission "could end at any time, without warning" and that "nothing was guaranteed about remission." The informants wondered why some cancer "seems to retreat" while another advances. Recurrence caused the informants to prepare themselves for the potential death of their wives: "I am hardening myself to accept the fact that she might not be here. I cannot say that I am giving up because we keep fighting every day."

Often, chemotherapy was viewed as "magic medicine" and was no longer feared because "it gave my wife years longer than we expected her to have." One informant thought his wife was coming out of remission and was told by a nurse that "it's a lot harder to get into remission the second time, and even if you do, it does not usually last very long." He could not bring himself to tell his wife and he carried the burden of this information alone. All of the informants in this study expected that "someday" the cancer would not be controlled. Although each recurrence was different, the informants went through the same process each time:

> I don't see how you could learn anything about how to control your emotions or how you are feeling. You are going to feel what I feel, absolutely devastated, no matter how many times you go through it.

> It's not something you ever get used to, that is, in the sense that it would be easier the second time around. I'm human, I'm not a machine. I'm not dealing with mechanical duplication only, I'm also dealing with emotions. You can't get used to that emotion so that you can handle it a little better the second time around.

> If you felt a certain way the first time around, it's not going to be easier just because you have been there once. You can't say I've been through it once, so the second time is easier. Could even be the second time is harder because now you are a person who has a tendency to preconceive the facts as they were.

Once a success had been achieved, however, the informants became more committed to *being positive,* hopeful, and living day-to-day:

> As her treatments worked, we would recognize it working. We would say let's not get morbid, let's stay alive, let's stay alert. We'll keep going. We'll keep making plans.

The attitude that "we will deal with that when we come to it" remained because the informants did not want to ruin "today."

At this point, there was a different emphasis placed on the phases of enduring: "We're just over the shock again, and getting back into the fighting mode. We are trying to talk about it a lot and face the facts." Also, during this time the diagnostic tests were not as important, for example one informant was not as aggressive about getting results because he dreaded the results and wanted to avoid *facing the fact.* Another informant, whose wife was afraid of the results of the diagnostic tests, went to get the test results alone. Taking the results home to his wife was difficult because they had always received them together.

The informants emphasized *orienting to the future* and *being positive* more than before the recurrence. They considered "what is it going to be like without her," especially when children were present in the family. One informant became less committed, decreased his help, and withdrew into himself, whereas other informants remained committed to their wives.

Emotions were close to the surface and the informants recognized their need to let them "overflow" when by themselves. The stress was incredible while the informants waited for test results and for physicians to determine "how to fight" and whether to initiate treatment. Trust in the physician's judgment was crucial to the informants' emotional adjustment. They needed to feel confident and secure in what the physician said about treating the disease with chemotherapy.

Talking about dying was taboo: "I never wanted to admit it, but deep down I did. We never talked about it." One informant, whose wife became progressively sicker, remembered questioning the efficacy of the treatment. His wife had given him her chemotherapy schedule, and he replied, "I don't think we are going to go." She told him, "you have nothing to say about this." He felt rebuked and guilty and after that he learned to disguise his feelings. Another informant whose wife endured repeated chemotherapy said, "I worried at home or whenever we were together. We did not talk about it, but it was constantly on our minds."

Several factors influenced the informants' abilities to implement strategies. These included the number of recurrences, the length of time between recurrences, and the length of time the disease had been progressing. As the length of the cancer experience and the frequency of recurrences increased informants found it more difficult to remain positive. They became more introspective when the physician or the wife did not appear to have a positive attitude about controlling the disease. During this time the informants were grieving while trying to maintain the facade of *being positive.*

The informants began conserving energy because they were afraid their wife was dying. They wanted to be ready to deal with the crisis of death. They began to wonder what it would be like, and they began thinking of plans they might have to initiate after their wife died. They were ambivalent about secretly getting ready, but they knew they had to *resist disruption* if they were going to be helpful. While the informants were afraid their wives were dying, they also felt guilty as they tried to make concrete plans: "Maybe I shouldn't be thinking about these things." Negative thoughts prevailed, and they worried about "becoming more positive": "I don't know how I would be able to handle it if I was all by myself, if my wife was not able to keep fighting." They did not want to think about this until they had to, but they found that this was almost impossible to do: "I was worried about my wife dying. I thought about how I would cope." Many of the informants coped by *keeping busy* and by helping others endure the battle. Other informants said their feelings changed for the better due to the personal strength they had developed to overcome this "horrible experience." Unfortunately, the informants never resolved "why" their wives had to go through this "punishment," and many of them believed chemotherapy was worse than the disease.

One of the concrete strategies the informants used was gathering more information. When acquiring knowledge they depersonalized the illness, which helped them to control their emotions in the presence of their wives. The initiation of treatment and the establishment of the treatment routine offered security, and the hope inherent in either the initiation of treatment or in the continuation of treatment offered longevity and enhanced *being positive*. *Being positive* was related to how one lived life and what was done to resist giving up, although being hopeful was related to the attitude one had toward controlling the disease and longevity. Thus one could be positive without being hopeful, but it was difficult.

The informants feared giving up the fight because they did not want to lose their wives, and they believed this loss would be "absolutely and completely devastating." They feared watching their wives suffer and die. They feared for themselves and the "emptiness" they would feel. They feared for their families and how they would manage. And their greatest fears were the loss of hope and the loss of *being positive* because they were afraid their wives would notice and be adversely affected.

Summary

The experience of husbands whose wives undergo chemotherapy is best understood as a three stage process: identifying the threat, engaging in the fight, and becoming a veteran. Throughout this process the husbands engaged in buffering behaviors designed to be protective and supportive. *Buffering* is a process with which the husband deliberately assesses actual or potential harm to his wife and then cognitively plans and implements strategies designed to buffer and maintain the wife's well-being.

Identifying the Threat

The total shock, fear, and loss of control associated with cancer was devastating for the informants in this study. The wait and watch approach used by some physicians caused the informants to feel helpless. Gaining control was the paramount strategy used to deal with the cancer experience, and the informants found themselves entertaining thoughts of *guarded optimism*. The informants did not want to oppose the wishes of their wives or the physicians, but they experienced doubt about their wives' ability to live with cancer. The buffering process began as the informants worried that their wives would sense the depth of their sadness and the doubt and uncertainty they had about the outcome of the cancer experience. The informants described mirroring their wives' anxiety and it is clearly evident from this study that the informants experienced stress in this life-threatening situation.

The informants began waiting, but the emphasis in this stage of the process was on responding to the confirmed diagnosis of cancer. They desperately tried to gain control by acquiring knowledge and making sense of or rationalizing the situation. The helplessness the informants felt was often expressed as anger.

Engaging in the Fight

Accepting the diagnosis and deciding to fight provided the informants with a sense of control. They believed they could help, but *guarded optimism* was always present. They were afraid to be too hopeful and compensated by becoming obsessed with the struggle to endure their wives' chemotherapy. During the fight, the desire of the informants to exhibit self-control and some measure of situational control was an underlying theme. As the informants struggled to buffer their wives from the effects of chemotherapy they also struggled to maintain control of their own feelings of helplessness. Being kept *in the dark* and the informants' perception of the lack of communication with their wives and with health care providers increased their feelings of helplessness and powerlessness. In most cases the informants had to learn to accept the lack of control and devise strategies to accommodate this situation.

To some degrees, sadness and fear were always present. With their ability to defer their emotions and focus on buffering, the informants displayed tremendous self-control. They assumed a passive role, especially when the effects of chemotherapy were dramatic. While this role had a buffering function, it also allowed the informants to hide their suffering. Although the informants only discussed issues related to dying when their wives introduced such topics, they certainly thought about their wives' deaths. A conspiracy of silence surrounded dying as neither spouse initiated or discussed the worst scenario related to cancer. The *doer* role helped the informants focus on their wives and reduced the stress caused by high expectations and guilt.

Several factors were potentially debilitating for the informants. They were overwhelmed by compassion and empathy for their wives, and in most cases the marital relationship became closer and stronger. Along with this the informants' sense of responsibility increased self-expectations, and this stressed the informants to the point where they were afraid of disappointing their wives or not being equal to their wives' admirable response to the chemotherapy treatment. The informants constantly fought feelings of guilt created by being the healthy bystander watching the effects of chemotherapy. Their wives' mood swings and nausea were the most disturbing emotional and physical effects for the informants to endure, and the lack of socializing and loneliness were frequently mentioned as adverse effects on their life-style. Part of the loneliness was self-inflicted as the informants rarely shared their concerns, feelings, or emotional responses with anyone. They spent the majority of their time working or at home, and they were left to engage in solitary events when their wives were ill or sleeping.

In order to acquire control, for example to make appropriate decisions based on adequate knowledge, the informants felt they had to be knowledgeable about the kind of cancer their wives had and the progress of the cancer growth. Their ability to cope depended on the information they were able to acquire. Often, due to the attitude of the health care providers, and their wives, the informants' access to information was blocked and sometimes completely refused.

The informants in this study planned and implemented many coping strategies. Strategies functioned as buffers, for example those designed to *soften the blow* or *resist disruption*. Without the maintenance strategies included in *preserving self,* the buffering process would have been ineffective. The informants recognized that these behaviors were a source of strength, but their ability to talk with others about their anger, fears, and concerns appears to have been detrimental to their ability to adapt to this stressful situation. The informants may have overcompensated with *keeping busy* and focusing on their wives in order to deny these feelings, but the feelings always came back to haunt them during quiet moments. Some of them wished they had been able to talk to someone else, particularly an outsider, and they recognized that remaining silent had impeded their ability to cope with the cancer experience. Denial and living for today seemed to be the essential ingredients in *being positive. Being positive* was the basis for their day-to-day lives and it revealed an effort to overcome the paradox of *guarded optimism. Being positive* incorporated trust and hope in the efficacy of chemotherapy; unfortunately, *being positive* was often enacted with considerable effort because of the constant awareness that the chemotherapy might not be successful in eradicating their wives' cancer.

Becoming a Veteran

Although the informants described relief and happiness when the chemotherapy was over, they were also doubtful and fearful about the progress of the disease. The perceived lack of positive feedback from health care providers had a detrimental effect on the informants. They had to continue to generate *being positive* for both their wives and themselves, and they experienced a serious lack of energy. Without the *doer* role to keep them physically active many of the informants felt lost. They had focused all their energy toward buffering and this changed as their wives became more independent. This change was disturbing and puzzling to the informants and they had to reevaluate their role. Anger began to be expressed. As the informants had been too occupied actually to think about the cancer experience, some felt this was the time of accepting the reality of their wives' cancer. Thus, in order to accept the illness it had to have a personal meaning for them, and this could not be determined without time, thought, and a less stressful environment. They needed to find something positive in the experience, and often this was reflected as a growth in themselves and in the way they saw the world around them. As they considered themselves experts, many of them wanted to become involved in helping others experiencing chemotherapy for cancer.

Recurrence

Recurrence restarted the process of identifying the threat, engaging in the fight, and becoming a veteran. Although better equipped, the total devastation and loss of control recurred when the cancer reappeared. Metastasis was feared because it was synonymous with death. Death was a topic that was never discussed and this was very stressful for the informants as they desperately tried to think positively and *second-guess* their wives' responses. Worry was evident but not discussed, and the informants began once again to wait for the test results which were pivotal milestones upon which decisions were made for further chemotherapy. It was a relief to begin chemotherapy again because it meant the cancer was being treated and hope was still alive. Although the informants became hardened to a future without their wives, they never totally accepted the idea. They did not feel as guilty thinking about the future because it was becoming a short-term reality. Perhaps because they had become so energy depleted and could not deny their own feelings anymore, the informants were more aware of their need to conserve energy. They were forced to step out of their long-standing strategy of living day-to-day and *being positive,* and they became vulnerable.

Note

1. The sample consisted of 15 husbands, aged 32-65, whose wives were experiencing either new or recurring cancer which required chemotherapy. Informants were deliberately sought from the community by advertising for volunteers in newspaper articles and circulars. A total of 48 interviews and one diary were included in the data analysis. Interviews with nine of the informants were conducted by telephone, and the remainder were face-to-face. Six of the husbands' wives were undergoing chemotherapy at the time of the study; the remaining nine wives had completed chemotherapy treatments. Six of the wives were deceased at the time of study completion.

References

Fernsler, J. (1986). A comparison of patient and nurse perceptions of patients' self-care deficits associated with cancer chemotherapy. *Cancer Nursing, 9,* 50-57.

King, T., & Taylor, C. (1987). The outpatient way. *Canadian Nurse, 83*(9), 23-25.

Klagsbrun, S. (1983). The making of a cancer psychotherapist. *Journal of Psychosocial Oncology, 1*(4), 55-60.

7

Toward a Theory of Illness:
The Illness-Constellation Model

JANICE M. MORSE
JOY L. JOHNSON

Wellness is a state of optimal comfort that is disrupted by the occurrence of an illness episode. Although illness physiologically affects *one* individual, the experience of illness, and in particular a *serious* illness, can affect and involve the entire family and other significant people in the experience of suffering, pain, and threats to life. Consequently, illness may be viewed as a distressing and disruptive period during which the minimization of suffering and the attainment of comfort become paramount. Because the ramifications of illness extend suffering beyond the individual to the family and others, *attaining comfort* takes the form of any number of strategies used by the ill individual, by those who are close to the ill individual and who share the suffering, or as an interactive process negotiated by any number of individuals involved in the illness experience. The goal of those involved in the illness experience is to decrease the suffering of the ill person or the shared suffering, thereby increasing well-being.

In the literature there are two major conceptualizations of the illness experience. First, illness has been conceptualized as the individual's experience of symptoms, which has been extensively described as the *Medical Model* (see Figure 7.1). From this perspective the practitioner focuses on the individual and is *primarily* interested in the patient's report of physical symptoms as cues to underlying disease processes. A second view focuses on the *person* and considers illness behavior as the ability of the ill person to cope with or to respond to the disease process. For example, Lazarus (1966) viewed illness as a cultural, mental, and somatic stressor that

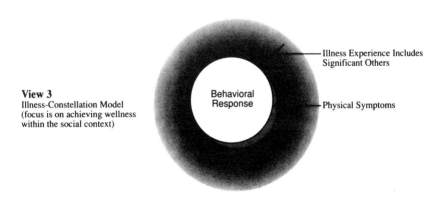

View 1
Medical Model
(focus is on physical symptoms)

View 2
Adaptation - Coping Model
(focus is on the illness behaviors)

View 3
Illness-Constellation Model
(focus is on achieving wellness
within the social context)

Figure 7.1. A Comparison of the Focus of the Medical Model, the
Adaptation-Coping Model, and the Illness Constellation Model

threatens bodily harm and disrupts motivational behavior. More
recently, researchers who use the phenomenological method have
viewed illness from this perspective (for example, see Kaufman,
1988). Thus this second conceptualization of the illness experience

is more complex because it incorporates not only the physical symptoms, but it also incorporates the human responses to these symptoms.

A more comprehensive view of illness, entitled the *Illness-Constellation Model,* has been developed by the authors. This model views illness as an experience that affects the sick person *and* his or her significant others. In this view, the ramifications of the individual's illness experience cause profound changes in the interactions, roles, and relationships of those involved in the illness experience and result in a loss of normalcy. Particularly in the case of serious illness there is an interplay of compensatory relationships between the sick person and his or her family and friends. The task of *regaining normalcy,* of regaining former roles and relationships with others is a legitimate task that must be resolved before the person regains a high level of wellness.

In the *Illness-Constellation Model,* the illness experience is defined as a four stage process. *Stage I* is the *Stage of Uncertainty,* and in this stage the individual detects or suspects signs of illness and attempts to make sense of these symptoms by determining their severity and meaning. Those closest to the ill person (usually family members and friends) observe that the sick person is unwell, but these observations may lag behind the experience of the ill person—or alternatively the ill person may have to inform others of the illness, for example in the case of a woman discovering a breast lump.

Stage II, the *Stage of Disruption,* begins when the individual makes a decision that the illness is real, is serious, and decides to seek help. This stage may also be initiated by the confirmation of a medical diagnosis or by the person suddenly becoming so ill that the decision to seek help is taken out of his or her hands by another person, for example taking the ill person to the doctor or calling an ambulance. This is a stage of crisis, a stage in which the individual relinquishes control and withdraws by *distancing* him- or herself from the situation. At this point the individual becomes totally dependent on health care professionals and family members. Significant others become aware of the illness and the threat it poses, and they may hover, be vigilant, and, as concerned friends or relatives, *suffer* with the individual. In the case of serious illness, relatives and friends assume the day-to-day responsibilities of the ill person, such as taking care of the ill person's children.

Stage III is the *Stage of Striving to Regain Self,* and in this stage the ill person *strives to make sense* of the illness. During this stage the ill person examines the past for reasons that explain the illness, and he or she tries to predict the future ramifications of the illness. Significant others find themselves *committing to the fight,* working and assisting with treatments and day-to-day tasks, and supporting and encouraging the individual. *Preserving self,* which involves conserving and focusing energy, becomes a priority for the sick person, while significant others engage in *buffering* behaviors, that is behaviors that reduce stimuli and protect the sick person from undue stressors. As the ill person is placed in a passive role, he or she must constantly negotiate and renegotiate with others in order to preserve his or her self-identity, control, and roles, and as he or she regains wellness, he or she must negotiate and prove to him- or herself and to others that he or she is well enough to resume tasks and responsibilities that have been assumed by others. Significant others who permit the ill person to be dependent and provide assistance with day-to-day tasks are hesitant to force the ill person to resume activities, yet they realize that although it is necessary for the sick person to relinquish some of his or her responsibilities and become dependent, total relinquishment on occasion may be harmful. The skill is to attain a balance or a reciprocal relationship in which the needs of both individuals are respected.

Frequently, this balance is attained by the sick person *setting goals,* and the attainment of these goals may indicate physiological improvement or a return to social functioning. While setting these goals, family and friends endure the illness process, policing and modifying the ill person's goals to ensure that they are realistic and attainable and providing necessary, realistic support and encouragement.

The last stage, *Stage IV,* the *Stage of Regaining Wellness,* is the stage in which the ill person *attains mastery* by regaining former relationships and the control of self. During this stage, the ill person determines when he or she is "better" or adjusts to and accepts a changed level of functioning. Family and friends assist the ill person in *making it through,* providing support and allowing the ill person to gradually regain control of his or her life. The ill person focuses on *taking charge,* learning to trust his or her body, to recognize and monitor symptoms closely, and to live within the new limits set by the illness.

Figure 7.2 summarizes the five studies included in this text and identifies the major strategies that were used by families and individuals in the various stages of illness. The stages and strategies of the *Illness-Constellation Model* (see Figure 7.3) were developed by synthesizing the findings of these five studies, eliciting the commonalities of each stage and comparing the main characteristics of each of the models.

In the following sections, the *Illness-Constellation Model* is discussed in detail in order to show how it affects both individuals and their significant others. As each strategy describes the ill person's response, the equivalent strategy that describes the response of the family or friends will also be discussed. For example, in the *Stage of Uncertainty,* both the ill person and the significant others engage in suspecting, and this is listed as "Suspecting ↔ Suspecting." Next, the ill individual engages in Reading the Body, and the significant others engage in Monitoring. These strategies are listed in tandem as "Reading the Body ↔ Monitoring."

Stage I. The Stage of Uncertainty

Suspecting ↔ Suspecting

The illness experience commences as the individual begins to *suspect* that something is wrong. They note that things are not quite right—their periods are irregular, they seem more stressed, a "funny feeling" of nausea overtakes them, they lose their appetite, or they find a lump in their breast—and confronted with these symptoms, the individual begins to suspect that something is wrong:

> I thought, "Gee, should I stop for lunch or shouldn't I? . . . I didn't have any breakfast today, maybe I'm feeling a bit hungry." So I made myself a half a sandwich. I normally make a whole sandwich, and I thought, "I wonder why."

Family and friends may also note behavioral changes in the ill individual or they may be directly told by the ill individual about

Author				
Johnson	Chassé	Lorencz	Norris	Wilson
Defending Oneself • Normalizing Symptoms • Struggling to Maintain the Status Quo • Distancing Oneself ↓ **Coming to Terms** • Facing One's Mortality • Making Sense • Facing Limitations • Looking to the Future ↓ **Learning to Live** • Preserving Self • Minimizing Uncertainty • Establishing Guidelines for Living ↓ **Living Again** • Accepting Limitations • Refocussing • Attaining Mastery	**Experiencing a Disruption** • Experiencing Symptoms • Learning to Read the Body • Negotiating Medical Management ↓ **Struggling to Preserve Wholeness** • Observing the Changes • Managing the Separation • Becoming a Patient ↓ **Recovering** • Adjusting to Changes • Coming to Terms	**Being a Failure** • Not Making It • Being Overwhelmed • Getting Admitted ↓ **Being in Boot Camp** • Planning for Goal Attainment • Gaining Control • Assessing Readiness • Getting Out ↓ **Anticipating Mastery** • Becoming Ordinary	**Suspecting Pregnancy** • Informing • Assessing Sexual Activity • Monitoring • Being Vigilant ↓ **Taking Responsibility** • Considering Alternatives • Consenting • Waiting ↓ **Reconciling the Abortion** • Grieving • Seeking Closure • Assessing the Outcome ↓ **Recovering** • Putting it Behind	**Identifying the Threat** • Suspecting • Finding Out ↓ **Engaging in the Fight** • Resolving • Inducting • Enduring • Finalizing ↓ **Becoming a Veteran** • Making it Through • Recognizing Changes • Marking Time

Figure 7.2. The Stages of Illness as Described in Five Grounded Theories

suspicious symptoms. In turn, family and friends also are drawn into the process of *suspecting*. Doubts begin to creep into the minds of the individual and family members as they grapple with the idea that something serious may be happening.

Reading the Body ↔ Monitoring

The symptoms experienced by the ill individual may begin insidiously and slowly, and the question the person asks about each subtle change is *Is this normal?* For example, in Chassé's study, women tolerated increasingly severe dysmenorrhea, watching their periods to see if this one would be heavier than the last, to see if the

Illness-Constellation Model	
Self	**Others**
Stage 1: The Stage of Uncertainty	
• Suspecting	• Suspecting
• Reading the Body	• Monitoring
• Being Overwhelmed	• Being Overwhelmed
Stage 2: The Stage of Disruption	
• Relinquishing Control	• Accepting Responsibility
• Distancing Oneself	• Being Vigilant
Stage 3: Striving to Regain Self	
• Making Sense	• Committing to the Struggle
• Preserving Self	• Buffering
• Renegotiating Roles	• Renegotiating Roles
• Setting Goals	• Monitoring Activities
• Seeking Reassurance	• Supporting
Stage 4: Regaining Wellness	
• Taking Charge	• Relinquishing Control
• Attaining Mastery	• Making it Through
• Seeking Closure	• Seeking Closure

Figure 7.3. The Stages and Focus of the Illness Constellation Model

pain was increasing in severity, or if the menstrual flow was normal or heavy. Each person begins *reading their body* by using their own past experiences to evaluate the present symptoms and, when the uncertainty continues, by comparing their own symptoms with their friends' experiences with menstruation. Chassé referred to this process as *establishing the boundaries of normalcy*. Similarly, in Johnson's study of heart attack victims, although the illness onset was necessarily more acute, all of the informants tried to evaluate the seriousness of the symptoms and to place the symptoms within the boundaries of known, familiar, and more common but less serious illnesses. At the onset of the heart attack these individuals tried to explain their symptoms as "the flu" or "something they ate." One informant, who had the classical signs of heart attack listed on a book mark, still did not interpret his symptoms correctly. Yet all of Johnson's informants were surprised at the fuss, speed, and sense of urgency their symptoms created when they finally consulted a doctor or reported to the emergency room. Were these people expecting heart attack symptoms to be more painful or more dramatic? Or did they not seek help, as Johnson suggests, because they preferred to remain in control and to regard their symptoms as trivial? The flu or the upset stomach was considered such a trivial complaint that these individuals would rather avoid the embarrassment of "troubling the doctor" than have their fears alleviated:

> I only had a slight idea what might be happening, but I thought the standard "Hey it can't be me." So I got up and threw up once. I was getting weaker all the time. But I stayed at work for the day.

In order to accurately read their bodies, ill individuals begin to identify *triggers* or situations that stimulate an attack or worsen or alleviate the symptoms. Again, in Chassé's study, this occurred frequently and over a long period of time before the women accepted the fact that their periods were abnormal and that they should seek medical help.

This process of normalizing symptoms is not limited to physical symptoms; emotional states are evaluated as well. For example, in Lorencz's study, the informants complained about increasing loneliness, problems with interpersonal relationships, and problems remaining employed, but again, one thing was clear: they saw themselves as "not making it" and of needing some help.

It is important to note that others also observed the sick person; *monitoring* the ill person for symptoms or assessing their level of wellness. In Norris' study, the mothers did this as soon as they suspected their daughters were involved in sexual relations, observing their daughters for signs of pregnancy:

> I've kept this to myself, but being a mother who washes her daughters' clothes, I do know when they have their monthlies. And I noticed that [daughter] didn't have anything on her clothes. It flashed through my mind [that she was pregnant]. . . . I certainly didn't want to believe it.

Similarly, Wilson reported that her informants monitored their wives over an extended period of time in order to determine what was happening to them.

Being Overwhelmed ↔ Becoming Overwhelmed

Eventually, the symptoms develop to a point where the individual is *overwhelmed,* both physically and emotionally, by a sense of uncertainty. Perhaps the process of deciding when you are sick *enough* to need a doctor is easiest when the symptoms are so severe that there is no question that medical help should be obtained immediately or when the situation is taken "out of the sick person's hands." The state of limbo, of the patient's not feeling well and yet not being sick, may be so stressful that receiving an actual diagnosis, the confirmation of being sick and the relief of an intolerably ambiguous situation, may be almost a relief:

> It's the unknown, the not knowing, which is the most stressful. It's fear of the unknown; fear of your mind starting to go off in all directions. You imagine all kinds of things.

On the other hand, the confirmation of malignancy (for example, finding a breast lump) may be devastating. The way the diagnosis is received by the patient depends on the severity of symptoms, the type of disease and prognosis, and the course of the illness.

If physicians dismiss the reported symptoms and do not provide the expected care or if they suggest unacceptable treatments or surgery the patient begins to "doctor hop," consulting one doctor after another. Chassé notes that her informants said many physicians did not give them information when requested, and in many encounters her informants were not treated with empathy and respect. Despite the fact that they were reporting severe and quite disabling symptoms they felt the physicians treated their complaints as "all in their head," and because they felt that they were not being taken seriously they were not in a position to negotiate treatments. If the patient's spouse is supportive during this time, this support adds weight or credence to the suspicion that something is *really* wrong, and the process of seeking medical help is eased considerably for the individual.

As family and friends witness the ill individual seeking medical assistance the fact that their relative or friend is ill becomes a reality. Often the friends and relatives *become overwhelmed* by worry and concern, particularly if they detect that the individual concerned is worried. Apprehension begins to grow during this waiting period, particularly if it is necessary for the ill person to undergo tests to rule out serious complaints. They vacillate, one moment considering the possibility of a devastating disease and the next moment reassuring themselves that such bad news is unlikely:

Waiting for results from the lab was really a torture situation. It was extremely stressful when you suspected very strongly, and yet nobody [will] come out and [say] this is what it is. When you're waiting for the phone to ring, you're wondering. It was very stressful waiting to hear. You felt so damn helpless. Phoning didn't seem to help. Nothing seemed to help.

Stage II: Stage of Disruption

The *Stage of Disruption* begins when the individuals realize that medical intervention is required and they no longer have a choice about whether or not they can manage their symptoms alone: either the symptoms are too severe, or the uncertainty is unbearable. A critical point is reached whereby either the person (or if they are unable, their relatives) transfers the responsibility for decision making to the physician.

Relinquishing Control ↔ Accepting Responsibility

Once the sick person enters the medical system, he or she no longer *really* makes decisions: choices become a medical prerogative. Rather than presenting alternatives for the patient to select or allowing the patient to decide whether or not treatment will even be instigated, the physician presents the selected course of treatment. Several factors contribute to the *relinquishing of control* on the part of the patient. First, in the physician-patient relationship the physician is often viewed as expert and the patient as the follower of expert advice. Second, urgent situations often necessitate the relinquishment of control, either because immediate action on the part of the physician is necessary or because the patient is not considered competent enough to make an informed decision. This lack of competence is exacerbated because of symptoms such as pain because the patient is not considered knowledgeable enough to make an informed decision, and perhaps because the patient is seen as a "case" rather than as a *person.*

This sense of lack of control is also felt by the family. For example, although the mothers and daughters in Norris' study had received permission from the Therapeutic Abortion Committee to have an abortion, they had difficulty grasping the fact that the abortions were *actually* going to take place, that the nightmare would soon be over. Similarly, Wilson notes that following the diagnosis for cancer her informants "were overwhelmed by the speed with which things happened." Once told about the diagnosis, these informants were pushed "from the frying pan to the fire, pretty quick," and they felt the necessity to receive immediate treatment. They felt *thrust* into a new situation, and there was "nothing they could do about it." This sense of immediacy was accelerated because they had an image of the cancer cells multiplying exponentially on a daily basis. Patients in this situation feel they have no choice but to trust the decisions of the physician. When a suspected heart attack victim experiences emergency care, the speedy response of health professionals is legendary. The patients are not active participants in their treatments; rather, they are viewed as objects who "have things done to them." Perhaps the most extraordinary description of this phase is from the psychiatric patients in Lorencz's study:

And the, all of a sudden, wham, I'm stuck in the hospital, and I was changed . . . and then the doctors got at me, and I was changed. I was—I didn't—I didn't give a damn for a while, eh? And the, and then, it got harder, even harder. And then the doctors got at me, and that's where I'm at. The doctors are talking about me, eh? What they think I am, and what they think, feel I want, and what I—do, and what I think, and stuff like that.

Seeing the vulnerability of the ill person and his or her inability to make decisions or to take control, the family and friends feel compelled to *accept responsibility* for them. Family members feel that they must "keep it together," not giving in to their own feelings of being out of control because they feel a sense of responsibility to act for their family member:

It reinforced for me that I'm here because I want to be here. She still is my daughter and my little girl. I wouldn't want to be anywhere else but here, and I am taking responsibility for her and for her error.

The family and friends' sense of responsibility is derived in part from the fact that they are healthy and their friend or family member is sick. Family members feel obliged to help in any way. They complete small tasks such as notifying others by phone and fetching basic articles for the sick person even though they are exceedingly worried and concerned. These small tasks keep them busy and help to relieve their anxiety. Consequently, helping is a comforting strategy. As one informant in Wilson's study indicated, "If you want to survive the situation, you really have to turn yourself into something that can be helpful to the person that's sick."

Distancing Oneself ↔ Being Vigilant

The loss of control requires total relinquishment of self on the part of the patient. In order to cope with the situation, they begin to *distance themselves*. Patients describe this as feeling as though they are automated; once begun, it seems that treatments cannot be stopped. As recipients of treatment ill individuals have little input into the decision-making process, and often they do not even know what is happening to them or who their doctor is. Often patients complain that things seem foggy, unreal, and that they have trouble grasping what is happening to them:

> Afterwards, it didn't seem like I had a heart attack. It didn't seem real. I thought, "Somebody else had it." It was funny. And it was kind of interesting. I thought about the fact that I had a heart attack, and it seemed almost impossible. It was like my brain didn't want to accept it.

During this time, relatives are *vigilant,* and although recognizing that their ill relative is unable or unwilling to take full control, they wait in the periphery in case they are needed or wanted. They struggle to get information, to understand what is happening, and to learn about the ramifications and outcome of the illness. Being vigilant often involves long periods of waiting and these waiting periods seem endless to the relatives. The family and friends feel that they must become the ill person's eyes and ears, trying to pick up whatever information they can in order to protect the sick person:

> You had to change your life-style a whole bunch. On those days, you obviously couldn't plan on going out. You had to be around to take care of your wife.

The patient in turn realizes the seriousness of the situation by the fact that the family is watching over him or her. The drain of knowing their family is waiting affects the sick patient, and this waiting increases their concern: "I was tense, she was tense. She got tenser from me, and I got tenser from her. We just kind of went around in a circle for a while." A patient in the ICU reported seeing her children "come off" the elevator while "they [the staff] were working over [her]." Although her children could not get close enough to communicate with her, she saw fear on their faces. Thus it is clear that the concept of *being vigilant* adds credence to the fact that the illness experience is a shared experience, occurring within reciprocal, dynamic relationships.

The *Stage of Disruption* ends as the individual begins to gain a sense of what is happening to them. They no longer feel that everything is in a fog and they are able to regain a sense of reality and engage more actively in the treatment process. For some individuals this stage is terminated by an acceptance of the terrifying fact that something has gone terribly wrong. No longer is it necessary for the individual to relinquish all control to physicians and family. Realizing that they must take some responsibility for themselves, they move into the stage of *striving to regain self.*

Stage III: Striving to Regain Self

Making Sense ↔ Committing to the Struggle

The *Stage of Striving to Regain Self* begins when the individual comes to grips with the illness and the future ramifications of the illness. They attempt to *make sense* of what has happened by asking friends and relatives who are present for details about their admission, resuscitation procedures, how they behaved while in pain, and other incidents that they can barely remember. They may also seek information from staff members or ambulance drivers. They examine events leading up to the crisis, they replay the story in their minds, and they tell and retell events to visitors and others as a part of making sense and accepting their present situation.

Inherent in this stage is the well documented process of soul searching for the "real" reason that *they* were stricken with this illness. Some find "just" cause, for example cancer of the uterus caused by a long past illicit abortion or a heart attack caused by living too well. Others are unable to answer the question "why me?":

> I kept thinking about it for the first month after I got home. . . . Just going over in my mind "Why did this have to happen?" And then I'd sit and ponder over it.

Family members go through a similar process, asking why, blaming themselves, and taking responsibility for the illness. This was evident in Norris' study where mothers accepted responsibility for their daughter's pregnancy, feeling somehow they should have been able to prevent this disaster. They wondered if this could have been avoided if they had been more strict, educated their daughters more completely, or somehow ensured that their daughters were properly using birth control.

Ill individuals are also confronted with the fact that their lives have been irrevocably altered. Although they might regain former functioning, because of the illness experience they see themselves in a new light. The suffering inherent in the illness experience forces the individual and the families to reexamine their lives, appreciating the things they had often taken for granted. They confront their mortality and reexamine their values. For some this is a positive experience encouraging them to redirect their life goals; for example, by making their relationships with their families a new priority. For others, however, the crisis of illness is so devastating that the implications are beyond comprehension. The sense of devastation that results from this may lead to depression, marital conflict, and withdrawal. The fact that life is irrevocably altered by the illness experience is clearly evident in all of the studies. For example, Lorencz's informants recognized that they would not only have to deal with the trauma of hospitalization but also the stigma attached to being sent to a place for "crazies." Mothers consenting for their daughters' abortions realized that their perceptions of who their daughters were would never be the same. Women who had experienced a hysterectomy faced the fact that they would never be able to bear children again. Husbands faced the threat that cancer would eventually recur in their wives. The fact that lives were permanently changed by the experience was clear when Wilson's informants discussed their wives' struggles even though their wives had died years ago.

Often any attempt by the relatives to make sense of the crisis is short-lived as they believe they should not focus on themselves but should commit all of their efforts toward helping their ill family member. For example, Wilson described how husbands had to "get it together" so that they could *commit* to the care of their wives. Thus while the individual is trying to make sense of what has occurred the family and friends are beginning to look to the future and are committing to the struggle that remains ahead.

Preserving Self ↔ Buffering

The immediate need of the person who is ill is the desire to regain control and preserve self. This is particularly difficult in the hospital environment as ill individuals are stripped of all responsibility and decision making, sometimes even of when and how to breathe. For example, they have to cough on command (even if it hurts) and they cannot go to the bathroom when they wish, choose their own meals, or eat whenever they want. Being unable to make even the simplest, most basic decision is demeaning and threatens the person's self-identity. Furthermore, removal from the home environment and the work place removes the cues that make one a unique individual and that give life purpose. The statement "Don't worry I've taken care of it" does not placate; instead, it increases the feelings of alienation and uselessness.

In order to *preserve a sense of self* the ill person begins to assert him- or herself and to reclaim control. They question treatment ("What's this pill for?"), and they seek information about their diagnosis, test results, and prognosis. They attempt to alleviate the signs of distress in their relatives' faces by trying to appear cheerful ("much better") and making light of their illness in order to minimize the concern demonstrated by their visitors:

> So they're [the informant's children] watching [the cardiac monitor]. They think they're going to get me excited, and I'm going to drop dead or something. So one day I looked up at it, and as I'm twisting to look up, I noticed it all went funny, and then I twisted a little more, and it went really funny. . . . So next time [my children came], I started wiggling around, and I said, "Hey, now watch that TV" . . . The older one said, "You're going to kill yourself. You can't do that." I said, "Oh yes I can. Watch this. Isn't it neat!" But you gotta have some fun or else you'd drop dead in there.

The relatives recognize that they must *buffer* and protect the ill person. They hover, attempting to shelter the ill individual from concern and worry:

> You do whatever you have to do for someone you love to make it as easy as possible. Everything I did was strictly for my wife. I had to do everything to make it easier.

The paradoxical nature of buffering is that it is done to protect the patient and allow the patient the time and energy needed to get well. If the buffering is excessive and too complete, however, they increase the sick person's stress as they sever the person from the

outside world and deny the ill person a sense of purpose. This
extreme buffering may become so protective that it retards recuperation and may even become disabling.

Renegotiating Roles ↔ Renegotiating Roles

Both individuals and their families must *renegotiate roles* and
responsibilities as the ill person recovers. Responsibilities are essential to the patient's sense of self and reclaiming former roles is the
major strategy used as the individual strives to regain self. Often ill
individuals attempt to regain a sense of control over their home and
work environments, even while still in hospital, by giving instructions, orders, and making decisions. Continuing to have input in their
"other lives" outside the hospital helps them to feel like human
beings rather than anonymous patients.

Once they return home ill individuals will often attempt to regain
a sense of sameness in the home so that the disruption of illness is
minimized. This was particularly true in Wilson's study when the
families contained children or in Norris' study where it was important
to maintain secrecy, when it was essential that the facade of normalcy was maintained. At this point patients are attempting to minimize the seriousness of their conditions by being cheerful and
reassuring their families, while the family members, on the other
hand, are attempting to coddle and reassure the patient. For the sick
person, maintaining normalcy by reclaiming roles minimizes the
impact of the illness and maintains the illusion that they are closer
to recovery than they are in reality. Although these people are sick,
somewhat dependent, and in need of help, the relatives must realize
that they need to allow the sick person, within limits, to give to them.
As one informant in Johnson's study said, "I think everybody needs
to be useful. If you have a feeling of being useless, I think you feel
what's the use of living sort of thing." Thus the relationship becomes
one of intricate interplay with the sick person, to some extent
concealing symptoms and negotiating in order to be treated as
"normal" while others observe for cues that suggest the sick person
is able to cope. Much like a dance, the sick person and the well
person accept and relinquish tasks. Recovery is not a linear process
but rather it depends on the resources of the sick person at any
particular point in time.

Setting Goals ↔ Monitoring Activities

It is important for ill individuals to believe that they will not remain ill forever. In order to feel that they are making progress, they often *set goals* for themselves. Accomplishing small goals such as walking a block or managing a stressful situation helps the individual feel that he or she is regaining control and is making progress in the struggle. In the case of the psychiatric patients in Lorencz's study, the schizophrenic patients worked to retain positive self-regard and planned for specific goal attainment. Because these individuals were not "making it" prior to their admissions they did not want to go back to the past but rather they were future-oriented, fantasizing about a normal life upon discharge:

> I'm gonna make a promise to myself that I'm gonna get out of that group home in ____ and get an apartment. And earn a . . . wage and eventually, eventually get back on my own and eventually earn my own keep, you know.

Meanwhile, family members are concerned that their relative might "overdo it," and they *monitor* the activities of the ill person, trying to ensure that they do not "push themselves" too hard. They chaperone, hover, and observe all the activities of the ill person, sometimes from a distance and always prepared to intervene if needed.

Seeking Reassurance ↔ Supporting

Throughout the *Stage of Striving to Regain Self,* a sense of uncertainty prevails, and the individual is forced to constantly *seek reassurance* from health care professionals as they strive for a sense of control. Seemingly trivial decisions, such as how much activity to engage in, when to regain sexual activity, or whether to lift a heavy object, are overwhelming as individuals attempt to manage their recoveries. It is only through a process of trial and error that daily routines are constructed to accommodate ongoing symptoms and fears:

> I'm still going through it, and I think, "Oh, I'm sure I can do this myself," and "Why can't I do it?" I'm scared of overdoing it. I'm worried whether I

should have a fear like that. I'm scared to do too much. And what is frustrating is I think, "Well, should I do it, or shouldn't I do it? Why do I have a fear of doing anything until I ask somebody if I can do it?"

Recognizing the uncertainty of their ill relative, family members engage in *supporting* the ill individual, giving them praise and encouragement and trying to instill in them a sense of hope. Family members offer support to the individual who is ill by making lifestyle changes, second-guessing his or her needs, reading about the illness, trying to remain positive (even if they do not feel positive), and by trying not to notice or comment upon the devastating effects of the illness.

Stage IV: Regaining Wellness

When the patients have once more regained a sense of self, they enter into the rehabilitative *Stage of Regaining Wellness*. This stage does not necessarily coincide with the patient's discharge from the hospital. The major tasks of this stage are regaining former relationships without the dependency of illness and once more asserting control over their own lives, learning to trust their bodies, putting the illness behind them, and attaining mastery.

Taking Charge ↔ Relinquishing Control

Relationships with friends and family members gradually return to resemble former patterns without the imbalance caused by the dependency that accompanies relationships when one of the partners is ill. Frequently the initiation of these changes comes from the rehabilitating person who is anxious to once again *take charge*. Often the recovering individuals feel that this is necessary in order to demonstrate their health and their competencies. For example, in Lorencz's study, patients felt they had to prove to themselves and to others that they were capable of surviving on their own after discharge. For other patients, this process of *taking charge* involved unwise actions:

I changed my living room around two weeks ago. My husband came home and just about shot me. . . . He said, "Good Christ, it's been that way for four years, it can stay that way." But I think it looks much nicer now, there's more room in it.

Often, dependent persons are anxious to take charge as they find the oversolicitousness of friends and family members to be both inappropriate and inhibiting:

> Well, there was a little anger building up in me because she's the oldest one, and she was the most protective. Like, I would get up out of my chair, and "No, no mom, don't. Where are you going? What are you going to do?" "I want to go to the bathroom." "Well, okay." And if I'd get up to do something, "No, no mom, no, no. You can't do that. No, no. Let me do it. Don't go upstairs again, oh no." And she'd be walking behind me and follow me up the stairs. I said, "I can go up and down the stairs twice a day, and that's all I do." I'd go to take a spoon out of the cupboard drawer, "No, no mom, sit down. I'll do that for you." Well, it just finally got to me. . . . So I just had to yell at her. And I yelled at her really good.

At other times the ill individual is forced into an independent role because of the demands of everyday living:

> Like the other day, he hit the corner of the heat register there and cut his little head open, and I mean, people say don't lift him up. But I think that was half my problem 'cause I lifted my son way too early, but they don't understand, like, how can you say no to a two year old?

As the ill individual begins to take charge, family and friends begin to *relinquish control*. This is possible because they see tremendous signs of improvement in the ill individual and are beginning once again to trust the ill individual's abilities and judgments. Seeing the ill individual return to activities such as lifting, driving a car, or returning to work reinforces the perception that the individual is once again able to care for him- or herself. Although some degree of monitoring may be maintained, it is usually done on a covert basis. If family or friends are unwilling to relinquish their control, ill individuals will increase their efforts to assert control over their own lives.

Attaining Mastery ↔ Making It Through

Throughout this final stage, ill individuals gradually learn to trust their abilities, and they work toward *attaining mastery*. They learn what their limitations are and how to extend their previous limits until they consider themselves well. Tentative trials of new physical tasks gradually give way to confident efforts:

> I'll tell you one of my happiest times was the summer after I had my heart attack. . . . We went to Banff, to Johnson Canyon . . . and we walked up the mountain there for hours. But I walked careful. I walked easy because I hadn't had my heart attack all that long ago. And I get to about four miles up there, hey, I felt great, and I thought, "God, I'm not a cripple." The last thing you want to be is a cripple. Nobody wants to be. A blind person doesn't want to be blind, and a deaf person doesn't want to be deaf, and a heart attack doesn't want to be a couch potato.

As small goals are reached and progress becomes evident, the overwhelming idea of rehabilitation becomes more manageable. Furthermore, "promotions" such as day passes and increased privileges for psychiatric patients facilitate the testing of the ill person's ability to make it in the "real world":

> By going through, going through the ropes, to use a cliché, I feel more comfortable having the approval of somebody professional saying, "When I started working in the snack bar, I felt more confident about being around more other people and being—putting myself in a social situation where the noise level and the conversation level was quite high—the potential for getting strained."

At this time the individual has to relearn the cues for reading the body, to learn when to become concerned over symptoms and the meaning of these symptoms. Perhaps because of the potentially serious ramifications of misreading symptoms and signs, this task requires a lot of energy and awareness. Constant comparisons are made with others or with one's previous state in order to determine if one is progressing and if symptoms should be a source of concern:

> I still got my same temper and everything, but something really has to happen to get me in a bad mood. Like before, it didn't take nothing. I just switched from one mood to the other with no reasoning, no nothing behind it, so that plays on your mind, too. You think you're going crazy.

The process of *attaining mastery* can continue for a prolonged period of time. Eventually, as confidence and a sense of control are gained, the individual is able to put the illness behind him or her and focus on other aspects of his or her life. A sense that he or she has regained wellness occurs gradually and becomes evident only when he or she realizes that he or she is no longer spending long periods of time being consumed by worry and concerns. Tasks are eventually completed without thinking twice about them, and the individual is able to put the illness experience behind.

As the individual works toward regaining mastery, family and friends focus on *making it through*. Although they rejoice in the victories of the ill person, they continue to be concerned about the future, unwilling to be convinced that the end of the illness is in sight. Often the family is concerned about reoccurrences. They do not want to become too enthusiastic about progress in case a set back is experienced.

Seeking Closure ↔ Seeking Closure

In this final stage, a major task that ill individuals and their family members engage in is that of *seeking closure*. Individuals cannot "get on with their lives" until they have satisfactorily resolved what has happened to them. For example, Chassé's informants said they could not move to a state of wellness until they resolved the question of whether they had made a correct decision when they had a hysterectomy. Those who were unable to affirm their decision to have a hysterectomy were unable to regain a feeling that their lives were back to normal:

> I feel so sad. I feel so empty inside, you know. . . . Towards my younger baby, I feel like I have to stick with her all the time. It's just an unbelievable feeling. I never felt that way before.

The family members also attempt to put the illness behind them. Although it is no longer a central concern, the poignancy of this experience, particularly the vulnerability of their partner, relative, or friend, remains with them. Having lived through the nightmare of an acute illness the family has a need to bring closure to the event. This desperate need for closure is expressed by a mother whose daughter had an abortion:

> I feel some kind of need to write closure to this, and I don't know how to do that. I should feel some sense of relief that it's over with, but there is so much pressure and tension and stress there that I have not been able to bleed it off effectively. . . . I am at a loss to know what it is that I need help with. I haven't identified that for myself yet. Like I know what it's not. . . . I can tell you what it's not, but I cannot yet tell you what it is. I am going to have to work this through.

Full closure, however, is never attained for the individual or for the family members. Heart attack victims continue to work hard to prevent another occurrence. Mothers continue to monitor their daughters' sexual activity to ensure that an unwanted pregnancy does not occur, and husbands vigilantly monitor their wives' health for signs of recurrence of cancer or metastasis.

Some individuals may be unable to return to a state of wellness following the illness experience. Failure to resolve the experience, the continuation of symptoms, and disability may all contribute to an inability to successfully put closure to the experience. Finally, it should be noted that the illness experience is not a simple linear process. Individuals experience "highs" and "lows" in this process, and some may return to previously completed stages several times. What does seem clear is that an individual will be unable to move on to a progressive stage until the previous one is complete.

Minimizing Suffering

In the *Illness-Constellation Model,* the core variable which underlies the entire process for both patients and their family and friends is *minimizing suffering.* The process of minimizing suffering consists of a variety of strategies directed at reducing the physical and psychological discomfort of illness, the social distress extending from changed roles and responsibilities, and the uncertainty of the unknown future. Suffering was therefore conceived to be a comprehensive concept incorporating the experience of both acute and chronic pain, the strain of trying to endure, the alienation of forced exclusion from everyday life, the shock of institutionalization, and the uncertainty of anticipating the ramifications of the illness:

> When you're thrown down into a pool, and you can't swim, and you don't have a life preserver, that's the way I felt for a long time. In other words, struggling. It was hard to get up in the morning knowing that you were going to have another one of those days which was unpredictable.

There is no doubt that the nature of the suffering experience has not been clearly described, and there is much work to do in the exploration of individuals' experiences as they cope and struggle with suffering in the illness experience. Furthermore, individuals do not suffer alone. The experience of suffering has ramifications for all those who are associated with the ill person:

> The pain of watching somebody that you love going through pain, going through agony, that is the hardest part. That is the hardest part of the whole thing to deal with that. That was my hardest part—it wasn't the caring or the cleaning up or the helping her to the washroom or getting the pills.

Because the nature of suffering incorporates physiological as well as psychological and social dimensions, *minimizing suffering* may be considered the *BSPPP* (a *basic social, psychological, physiological process*) in the *Illness-Constellation Model*.

Discussion

In this final chapter we have attempted to arrive at some general understanding of the illness experience. Clearly there is much research left to do before this complex process is fully understood. Although recent years have witnessed an increased interest in the experiences of those who are ill (Conrad, 1990), to date investigations have tended to examine illness by examining the individual's response to diseases. The bio-medical model is frequently used as a structure for understanding individuals' responses to specific diagnoses such as epilepsy (Scambler & Hopkins, 1990), Parkinson's disease (Pinder, 1988), or post partum depression (Harkness, 1987). Alternatively, researchers have focused on responses to specific symptoms, such as hypoglycemia (Hunt, Browner, & Jordon, 1990; Singer, Fitzgerald, Madden, Voight von Legat, & Arnold, 1987) or pain (Zborowski, 1969). Clearly, these investigations have offered valuable, *albeit* fragmented insights. It is ironic, however, to note that the medical model continues to be used to sample for behavioral theory. Perhaps the current fragmentation of illness theory is because of the *a priori* classification of behaviors based on medical diagnosis. Indeed, even the chapters of this book have been derived using this perspective of patients with medical problems. Attempts to move away from the medical model in illness theory need to be made, however. It is clear that there are commonalities in the illness experience that bridge the boundaries created by the disease taxonomy. These can be elicited just as Selye (1976) observed the physiological syndrome of "just being sick" many years ago.

Clearly, it is time to move on and develop a broader understanding of the illness experience using human behavior as a basis for developing theory. As the five studies included in this book have demonstrated there are remarkable similarities in the ways individuals and their families and friends live through and cope with the illness experience, and from these similarities the strength of the *Illness-Constellation Model* is derived. Although the *Illness-Constellation Model* overcomes some of the limitations of current illness theory in that it incorporates the experiences of individuals and their families and friends and is not limited to a single diagnosis, there is still much work to be done in this area. Instead of investigating illness as a series of discrete categories or isolated responses we need to further develop this Model and continue to investigate the illness experience comprehensively.

In particular, the role of the family needs to remain at the forefront of illness research. Too often the illness experience has been conceptualized as individualistic rather than reciprocal. Because of emotional ties, family and friends are intimately involved in and affected by the life of the ill individual and the impact that illness has on these individuals needs to be included. Another area that also needs to be considered is how individuals isolated from friends and family manage with their illness, particularly in Stage II of the

Illness-Constellation Model, the *Stage of Disruption.* In particular, the elderly are often without the support of family. How do these individuals' experiences differ from those with support systems? This area needs to be carefully investigated.

Another aspect of illness requiring careful consideration is the experience of those who do not recover from what is considered by medical personnel to be a recoverable disease. The plight of the "cardiac cripple" who is determined by a physician to be physically well yet is only able to function at a minimal level is a typical example of this phenomenon (Cassem & Hackett, 1977). There are countless examples of individuals who have suffered from a variety of diseases and are unable to regain wellness despite the fact that they have officially recovered from their disease. Conversely, there are individuals who remain physically disabled but reach a high level of wellness (Trieschmann, 1980). Both of these examples illustrate the inappropriateness of using medical diagnoses as the basis for examining illness behavior. Thus perhaps it is time to ignore the medical diagnosis and to use behavioral indicators when sampling for studies that are exploring behavior.

Suffering is inherent in the illness experience, particularly as these studies show in more serious illnesses. The experience of suffering may be short and intense or it may be a prolonged and insidious strain that "does not go away." The nature of suffering reflects the variable and often erratic course of illness. Yet despite the pervasive nature of suffering and the integral relationship of suffering and illness, this concept has been largely ignored in the research literature. There is a need for intensive investigation in this area.

In recent years, the focus of many qualitative studies has been on *chronic illness.* It is not clear to us, however, how chronic illness is differentiated from acute illness. Authors do not state if they use medical criteria or the criterion of duration to define "chronic," although we suspect it is the former. Nevertheless, when these chronic illnesses are examined from an experiential perspective their course is not dissimilar from that of acute illnesses. Perhaps the differentiation between acute and chronic illness represents a false dichotomy. There are similarities between the experiences of those who suffer an acute illness, those who suffer chronic illness, and those who may technically suffer from a nonillness, such as those who are undergoing abortions (see Norris, this volume). Certainly, the *Illness-Constellation Model* appears to fit acute and chronic patterns of illness. It appears that the "flare-ups" or exacerbations that occur in chronic illness are similar to episodes of acute illnesses. Furthermore, although a disease such as a myocardial infarction is officially classified as acute, the recuperative period is prolonged and the impact of this disease on the individual's life is permanent. At this point there is a need for further research to examine these chronic illnesses with a view to exploring further the acute-chronic differentiations.

Although the *Illness-Constellation Model* is not intended to expli-cate a "standard" response to the illness experience, it does provide important insights into how the ill individual and significant others respond to their situations. Clearly, variation in these experiences is expected and future investigation will enrich and explicate this model. Furthermore, this model is not intended to describe a linear process; rather, it is a process that may involve regression as well as progression. For example, individuals may progress to Stage III and later deteriorate to Stage II. Or as indicated in Wilson's study, cancer patients in Stage IV return to the *Stage of Uncertainty* (Stage I) as the individual suspects that the disease is recurring.

In 1984, Armstrong noted that the explication of the patient's view is not a recent innovation. Patients have always been expressive about their experiences. What is new is that we are beginning to listen more attentively and to give credence to the patient's perspec-tive. We are hearing the same stories but with new ears and with new research methods and we are gaining new insights. Our changing attitudes toward patient care places new value on the illness experi-ence as an important area of investigation. This refocusing of health care ensures that the patient is treated as a person, that the family is included in the care, and that the care is humane.

References

Armstrong, D. (1984). The patient's view. *Social Science & Medicine, 18,* 737-744.

Cassem, N. H., & Hackett, T. P. (1977). Psychological aspects of myocardial infarction. *Medical Clinics of North America, 61,* 711-721.

Conrad, P. (1990). Qualitative research on chronic illness: A commentary on method and conceptual development. *Social Science & Medicine, 30,* 1257-1263.

Harkness, S. (1987). The cultural mediation of postpartum depression. *Medical An-thropology Quarterly, 1,* 194-209.

Hunt, L., Browner, C. H., & Jordon, B. (1990). Hypoglycemia: Portrait of an illness construct in everyday use. *Medical Anthropology Quarterly, 4,* 191-210.

Kaufman, S. R. (1988). Toward a phenomenology of boundaries in medicine: Chronic illness experience in the case of stroke. *Medical Anthropology Quarterly, 2,* 338-354.

Lazarus, R. S. (1966). *Psychological stress and the coping process.* New York: McGraw-Hill.

Pinder, R. (1988). Striking balances: Living with Parkinson's disease. In R. Anderson & M. Bury (Eds.), *Living with chronic illness* (pp. 67-88). Boston: Unwin Hyman.

Scambler, G., & Hopkins, A. (1990). Generating a model of epileptic stigma: The role of qualitative analysis. *Social Science & Medicine, 30,* 1187-1194.

Selye, H. (1976). *Stress in health and disease.* Boston: Butterworths.

Singer, M., Fitzgerald, M. H., Madden, M. J., Voight von Legat, C., & Arnold, C. D. (1987). The sufferer's experience of hypoglycemia. In J. A. Roth & P. Conrad (Eds.), *Research in the sociology of health care: The experience and management of chronic illness, Vol. 6.* (pp. 147-176). Greenwich, CT: JAI Press.

Trieschmann, R. (1980). *Spinal cord injuries: Psychological, social and vocational adjustment.* Elmsford, NY: Pergamon.

Zborowski, M. (1969). *People in pain.* San Francisco: Jossey-Bass.

Index

About the Authors

Marie Andrée Chassé, RN, MN, obtained a Diploma of Nursing in 1979 at the Ecole de formation infirmière d'Edmunston and a BScN in 1983 at the Université de Moncton. She has recently completed a Master of Nursing at the University of Alberta. Her clinical experience includes oncology and medical/surgical nursing. She has several years of experience in nursing management, has been an assistant professor at the University of Moncton, New Brunswick, and has had a long-standing interest in women's health.

Joy L. Johnson, RN, MN, received her BScN degree from the University of British Columbia and her MN from the University of Alberta. Currently, she is a PhD candidate in nursing at the University of Alberta where she is engaged in a philosophic inquiry regarding the art of nursing. Her clinical experience has primarily been focused on the care of the critically ill adult.

Beverley Lorencz, BScN, MN, received her diploma in Psychiatric Nursing in 1976 from Alberta Hospital, Edmonton, Alberta. She worked for several years with the mentally ill and received her BScN (with distinction) from the University of Alberta in 1985 and her MN from the University of Alberta in 1989. Following graduation, she was employed as a staff nurse and head nurse (medicine) at the Charles

Camsell Hospital, Edmonton. She is presently employed in a small hospital in Northern Ontario.

Janice M. Morse, RN, PhD, is a Professor of Nursing, an Adjunct Professor in the Department of Family Studies and an NHRDP/MRC Research Scholar at the University of Alberta, and an Adjunct Professor at the University of Northern Arizona. With doctorates in both nursing and anthropology, her research interests focus on the experience of illness, in particular in the area of patient care and comfort. She has completed research on the topic of patient falls, infant feeding, childbirth, cross-cultural health, and has conducted fieldwork in Fiji. She has published more than 100 articles, has authored and co-authored several books, and is the editor of the journal *Qualitative Health Research*.

Judy Norris, RN, MSc, received a diploma in nursing from St. Patrick School of Nursing, Missoula, Montana, and BScN and MSc degrees from the University of Alberta in Edmonton. She has conducted qualitative research on mothers' responses to their adolescent daughters' abortions and (with Dr. Judith Hibberd) on nurses' experiences of working during a strike conducted by colleagues who belonged to another nursing union. Her areas of interest include nursing management research and staff nurses' life-styles and family issues.

Sharon Wilson, RN, MEd, MN, is a Professor of Nursing at Ryerson Polytechnical Institute, Toronto, Ontario, Canada. After receiving her diploma in nursing from Women's College Hospital in Toronto, she practiced nursing in an acute care setting and later began teaching nurses. Realizing her need for further education, she attained her Baccalaureate in Nursing degree at the University of Toronto, an MEd at Brock University, and a Master's Degree in Nursing at the University of Alberta. She has a strong commitment to excellence in nursing practice, and her teaching and research interests include surgical and oncology nursing as well as multicultural nursing.